MW01599180

PEGAN DIET

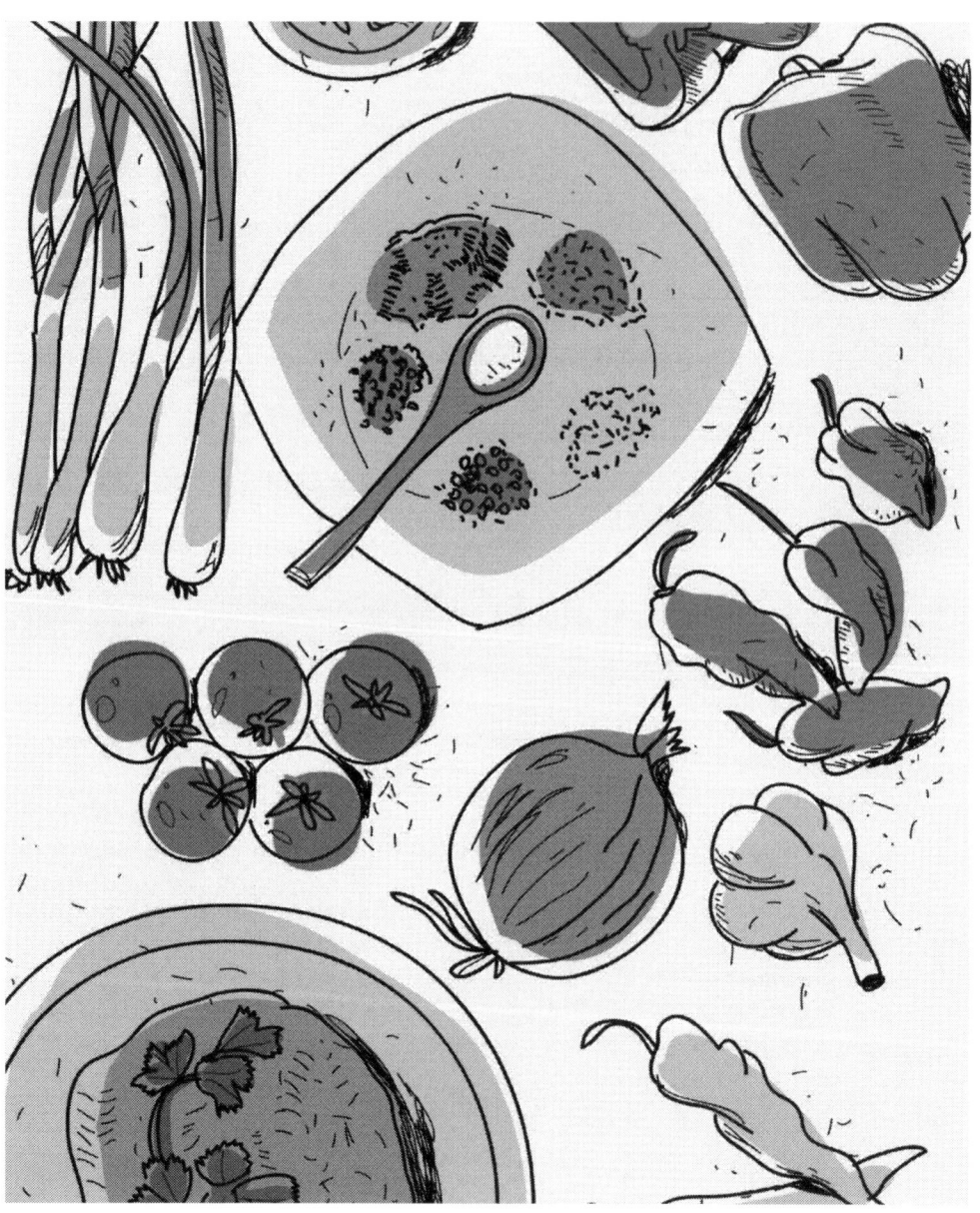

Pegan Diet

30 Day Pegan Meal Plan and Top 100 Pegan Recipes

Paige Russel

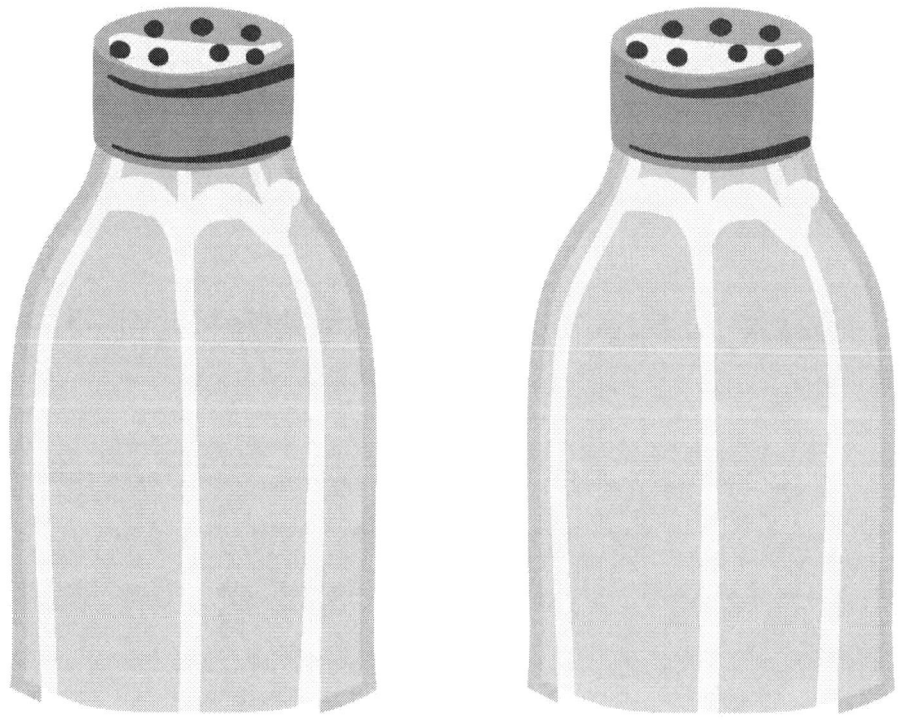

LEGAL NOTICE

Copyright (c) 2019 by Paige Russel

All rights are reserved. No portion of this book may be reproduced or duplicated using any form whether mechanical, electronic, or otherwise. No portion of this book may be transmitted, stored in a retrieval database, or otherwise made available in any manner whether public or private unless specific permission is granted by the publisher. Vector illustration credit: vecteezy.com

This book does not offer advice, but merely provides information. The author offers no advice whether medical, financial, legal, or otherwise, nor does the author encourage any person to pursue any specific course of action discussed in this book. This book is not a substitute for professional advice. The reader accepts complete and sole responsibility for the manner in which this book and its contents are used. The publisher and the author will not be held liable for any damages caused.

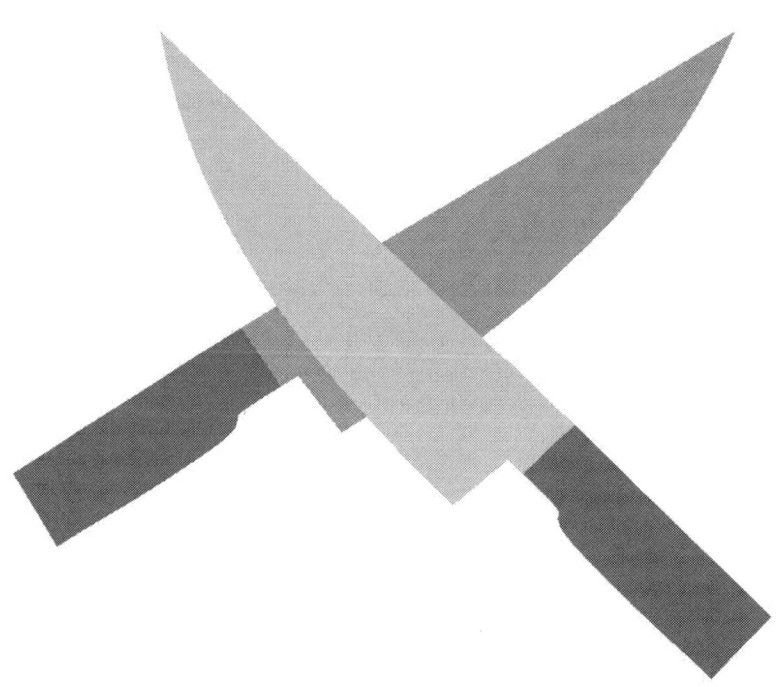

CONTENTS

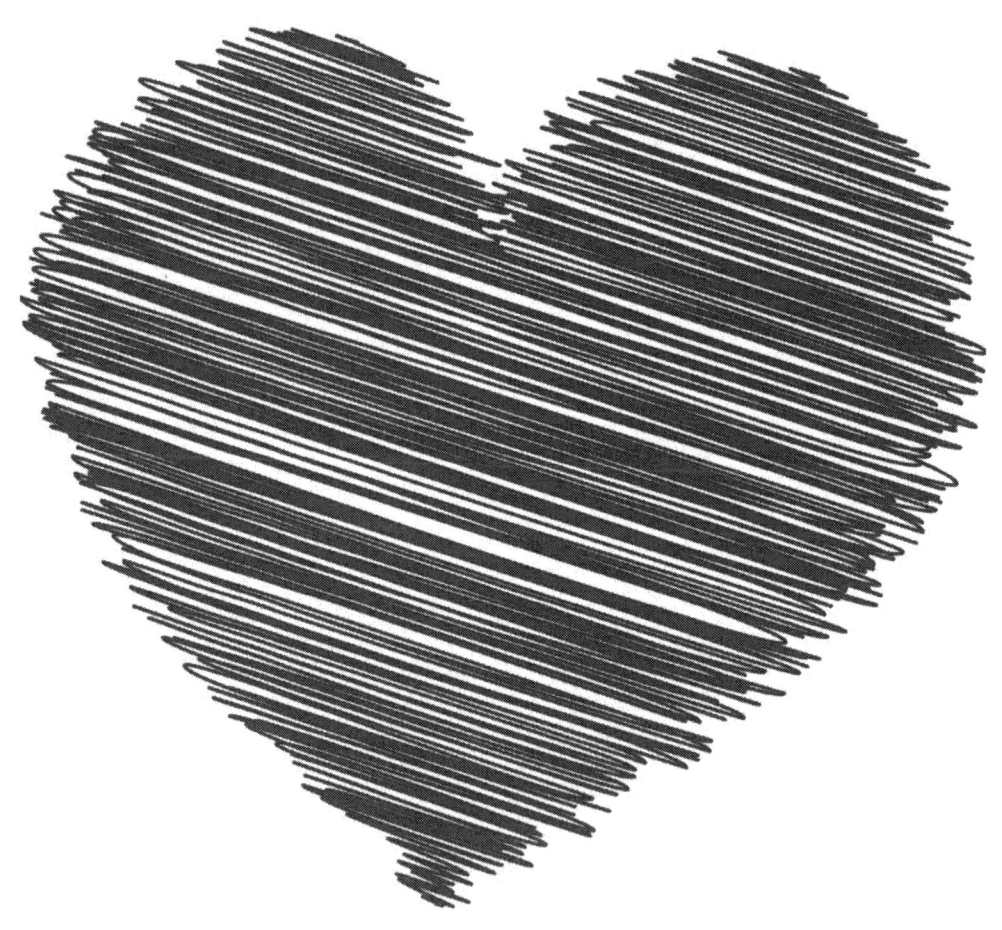

PEGAN DIET

WHAT IS THE PEGAN DIET?

Have you ever heard of the pegan diet? It sounds a bit odd, and evokes the idea of the vegan diet... or maybe the paleo diet? Well, true to what its name implies, the pegan diet is a fusion of sorts from both the paleo diet, and the vegan diet, seeking to combine the principles of both diets and try and get the best of both worlds. It may seem very strange, as paleo diet adherents are supposed to eat simple foods that were available in the paleolithic era millions of years ago, such as vegetables, fruits, nuts, fish, and meat, excluding dairy, grains, sugar, oils, and other similar products such as legumes, or even alcohol and coffee, as these were not around in those ages. The vegan diet, on the other hand, dictates that one strictly avoid animal products or byproducts, which includes meats, fish, eggs, cheese, and other similar products, requiring that one only eat plant based foods.

As such, one would be expected to be highly confused about the pegan diet, given its contradictory nature. However, what the pegan diet seeks to do is to combine certain principles from both diets, principles that will be discussed in – depth later. However, the general idea of the pegan diet is that one is supposed to eat nutrient – dense whole foods, which are able to reduce inflammation, balance blood sugar, allowing one to be at optimal health. As one would see that the pegan diet combines both vegan and paleo diets, both limited diets, one might think that this means that only the overlap between the two is allowed, which would result in a very, very limited diet indeed. However, contrary to this idea, it is even less restrictive than either vegan or paleo by themselves, as it seeks to combine principles, not the restrictions per se.

A lot of emphasis is placed on eating fruits and vegetables, like the vegan diet, but unlike the vegan diet, consumption of animal proteins such as meats and fish are allowed, as well as some nuts, seeds, and legumes. In fact, even some items that are banned by both are allowed, such as oils and some processed sugars, but note that these should be highly restricted. The pegan diet is not a crash diet, but rather a sustainable diet meant to be easy to stick to, which allows one to stay on it indefinitely rather than losing willpower to continue later on.

What are Pegan Diet Tenets?

Now that we have a basic idea of what makes up a proper pegan diet, we should look at the principles, or the tenets behind the pegan diet. These are tenets that one has to be aware of, as it may be a bit confusing to just use the rule of thumb. After all, a vegan diet is clear; one can only eat plant based things. A paleo diet is also fairly clear: one should eat simple, unprocessed foods. However, as a pegan diet is separate and distinct, and is actually less restrictive, the limitations and tenets are not as intuitive.

Focus on having a mainly plant – based diet

The first tenet is that one should mostly have a plant – based diet. Though as we stated earlier, consumption of animal proteins is allowed, the majority of the things one eats should be plant – based. In fact, a good rule of thumb to go by is half or a bit more than half of one's plate should be filled with vegetables at the minimum. About seven or eight cups of vegetables and fruits a day is the recommendation of the World Health Organization, and would serve as a great starting point. However, not all plant – based foods should be indulged in great quantities. Some foods, such as starchy vegetables like potatoes and squash should be more limited, with the majority of the vegetable portion being leafy greens instead. After all, one of the aims of this diet is to help regulate one's blood sugar, meaning that prioritizing low – glycemic index foods is important to the diet, and having foods high in simple carbohydrates, high glycemic – index foods would defeat the purpose. In addition, fruits are also something that should be limited, along the same principles behind the restriction behind limiting starchy vegetables. However, this tip is more for those who are still overweight, and have a greater need to manage blood sugar. If one has no blood sugar problems, most fruit is fine. If one is plagued with managing their blood sugar, however, mostly low – glycemic index fruits should be consumed, with sweeter fruits being a treat every so often, being treated more like candy rather than a regular part of one's dinner plate.

Make sure to consume healthy fats

The second tenet would be to aim mostly to consume healthy fats. Fats are a very important part of one's nutrition, but remember that it is best consumed in its whole food form. Some of these better fats would be found in unprocessed foods such as nuts, seeds, avocados, olive oil. Some animal products that have healthier fats would be eggs, and some fatty fish such as salmon, mackerel, herring, and sardines. Using extra virgin olive oil or avocado oil, or even coconut oil as a way to garnish uncooked dishes such as salads, or to use when cooking would help. Remember that as this is not a vegan diet, animal and saturated fat from unprocessed sources is allowed, such as from meats, fish, eggs, or even butter or ghee. Note however that saturated fat is very bad for you if it is combined with refined sugars and starches. In addition, common oils such as vegetable, bean, and seed oils tend to be very processed, and thus are not recommended to be used.

Consume Meat in Moderation

One of the most surprising things that people notice about the pegan diet is that it allows meat to be eaten, even if it takes a lot from the vegan diet. However, even if meat is allowed, it is recommended that it is kept to a small amount per meal, and in fact should act as more of a side dish or condiment, with the vegetables making up the majority of the meal. Note that there are also some forms of animal protein that can be consumed other than poultry or grass – fed beef, such as insects, though this may be only for the more adventurous souls.

Eat whole grains and beans

Make sure to include only whole grains in your diet, and ignore other types of grains. In fact, even grain flours should be avoided. However, when it comes to whole grains, these should still be limited to small portions, to about one cup maximum per meal. Even though some grains can have high protein content, the focus should still be on leafy vegetables. Beans are another good inclusion, but starchy beans should be avoided. However, lentils and other similar beans are good for you as they are great for introducing fiber, protein, and minerals in one's diet, though they should be cooked thoroughly in order to limit the amount of digestion problems that one may end up having thanks to bean consumption.

Avoid processed sugars

While sugar need not be totally eliminated from one's diet, processed sugars should be avoided as much as possible, as the pegan diet aims to steer us away from anything that could spike insulin production and elevate blood sugar. However, this does not mean one is banned from eating sugary things, but consumption should be extremely limited, and this should be seen as a treat, and not a regular item in your diet.

Limit Dairy Consumption

One thing people who end up adhering to the vegan diet or the paleo end up missing the most is dairy. Dairy products are one of the favorite products of people all around the world, and the fact that paleo and vegan diets limit this is one hump that a lot of people have a hard time getting over. In this case, with the pegan diet, dairy is permissible. However, thanks to the high impact dairy has on the environment, due to the production process, it is advised that it is to be consumed in limited amounts, and as much as possible, sourced from sustainable sources. However, dairy is a good protein source, and can be treated as such.

Avoid chemicals and preservatives

As much as possible, chemicals and preservatives should be avoided in foods. This includes chemical additives, preservatives, dyes, artificial sweeteners or other junk ingredients. GMO foods are all right, though as much as possible, natural foods are better. However, as GMO foods are meant to make production more efficient, with more food produced relative to land used, they are also helpful in improving sustainability, but GMO foods also tend to go through a lot of processing, so they should still be consumed in limited amounts.

Choose Sustainably Produced Foods

As much as possible, food that is consumed should be food grown sustainably, though this is more for the health of the planet and the environment more than personal health. As much as possible, organic, grass fed, and pasture raised meats should be used, and when it comes to fish, wild fish is always preferable, due to the less amounts of dangerous chemicals, such as mercury, but again, one must ensure that they were sourced sustainably.

HOW IS THE PEGAN DIET MORE COMPLICATED THAN SIMPLY PALEO + VEGAN?

As we have discussed, the pegan diet combines both paleo and vegan diets, aiming to take as many of the pros as possible, while limiting the cons. Here we examine the paleo and vegan diet pros and cons, and we see how they are balanced by taking the pegan diet.

Paleo and Vegan Diet Pros and Cons, and How the Pegan Diet Balances them

Vegan Diet Pros

Weight loss

One of the more popular health reasons that people go vegan is for weight loss. Given today's world, many people have become overweight due to over – eating and over – consumption of high – calorie food such as fast food and junk food, these being loaded with oil and sugars, particularly high – fructose corn syrup. As such, people have begun to turn to vegan diets in order to provide them with a healthy, low – calorie alternative to the fast – food or frozen food fads that are popular and convenient today. After all, it is only logical to think that vegan diets assist with weight loss, as the core principle behind losing weight is that the calories burned are more than the calorie intake, and the simplest way to achieve that is to reduce the number of calories that a person takes in. Vegetables and plant – based foods naturally have a far lesser number of calories proportionally as compared to meats and other animal products, meaning that for the same amount of food that a person eats, they will be taking in far less calories if they eat vegan as compared to an omnivore's or a carnivore's diet.

This theory is borne out in practice. Multiple scientific studies published in reputable journals such as *Nature* and *the American Journal of Clinical Nutrition* have concluded that vegans tend to have lower body mass indexes. Other studies have shown that dieters that wish to lose weight, tend to lose it faster when on a vegan diet. It is worth noting that while normally it may be attributable to other characteristics, such as a more active lifestyle, these studies control for these other external factors, and still come to the conclusion that vegan diets lead to greater weight loss.

One of the great things about this is that these people on vegan diets don't even have to necessarily feel like they are restricting themselves, as they are usually allowed to eat until satiation. This is where the low – calorie and high – fiber nature of most vegan diets kicks in, meaning that less calories are naturally absorbed, even given a high – volume of intake. The same volume of meat that may have resulted in a caloric intake of about seven hundred calories (700 kCal) may end up simply being worth two hundred calories (kCal) for the same volume of plant matter.

Improved Nutrition

In addition to losing weight, one of the great things about having a vegan diet is the fact that at the end of the day, your body tends to end up healthier; after all, weight and body mass index is not the only, nor even necessarily the best indicator of a person being healthy. Though it can't be seen on the surface, good nutrition is one of the best ways to stay healthy and fit. A person can look fine on the outside, yet have a lot of things wrong with them; they can be sick and unhealthy without looking like it. This only means that health should not merely be gauged through weight.

So why do vegans often enjoy better health than their counterparts? This is because of the better nutrition that their diet affords them. The abundance of nutrients in vegetables, such as potassium, magnesium, Vitamins C and E, just to name a few, helps in ensuring that the body has what it needs in order to maintain itself and keep itself healthy. This, in addition to the fact that vegetables are much higher proportionally in unsaturated fats (the good kind), as well as being naturally high in dietary fiber and low in cholesterol, means that eating vegetables tends to be far healthier for the body, as it doesn't have as many problems processing the food that is eaten.

One extremely important thing to note, however, is that while vegetables themselves contain a lot of essential nutrients, and in high enough proportions that the body will not lack for these particular nutrients, there are some nutrients that cannot be provided by an all – plant matter diet, such as Vitamin B – 12, vitamin D, calcium, and certain fatty acids such as the long – chain Omega – 3 fatty acid commonly found in fish, as these nutrients cannot be synthesized by the body, and must be taken in from an outside source, and the most bio – available source for humans is to get it through animal products. As such, vegans are recommended to supplement their diet using appropriate supplementation, in order to make sure that they get all the necessary nutrients to maintain their health, and to make sure that they keep a balanced diet.

In short, a vegan diet has a myriad of health benefits including improved nutrition, as vegetables and fruits are usually nutrient – dense. However, this comes with a caveat that plants cannot supply people with all of the nutrients that are necessary, so this must be made up for by taking proper supplementation.

Lowered Risk of Contracting Certain Diseases

Those with a vegan diet have a two – fold way of reducing the risks of type – 2 diabetes. First, they tend to shed weight and keep it off, a very effective way of helping the body deal with high blood sugar levels. Second, their diet, based off of plant – matter, has a tendency towards reducing blood sugar levels in the first place, due to their lower sugar content, as well as their high dietary fiber. In fact, it has been shown that in general, vegans have a seventy – eight percent (78%) lower risk of developing type – 2 diabetes, and the average blood sugar level of a diabetic that switches to a vegan diet has been noted to be up to two point four (2.4) times lower than other diets as recommended by the American Diabetes Association and the American Heart Association.

The benefits of a vegan diet in reducing a person's risk factor for disease is not only limited to type – 2 diabetes, but extends to one of the greatest killers in the world today: heart disease. Many studies have shown that vegans tend to have a quarter of the risk (75% lower) when it comes to developing high blood pressure or hypertension, one risk factor for heart disease, and an overall forty – two percent lower (42%) risk factor for heart disease to be the cause of death of vegans as compared to the general population.

There are also other diseases whose risks are reduced for those who have a vegan diet. One of them is cancer, where there is a fairly significant drop of fifteen percent (15%) for the overall risk of cancer of any kind. This is a significant reduction in risk, and has been attributed to the maintenance of a consistent vegan diet. Another disease that has a lower risk factor for vegans is kidney disease. Vegans and vegetarians showed improved kidney functions, such as an increase in their "GFR", or glomerular filtration rate, as well as a lower amount of creatine and urea, which means that their kidneys are functioning better, and have a lesser load to filter, as compared to those that have animal protein as a significant portion of their diet.

Some other diseases that have a reduced risk factor is Alzheimer's disease, a degenerative brain disease that often results in memory loss, dementia, and eventually death from complications. Studies have shown that there is a tendency towards a lower incidence (less occurrences) of Alzheimer's disease in vegans, controlling for age and genetic factors. Not only does a vegan diet reduce the risk of incidence of Alzheimer's disease, it also tends to show that those vegans that have Alzheimer's disease tend to have a delayed onset of dementia, which means that they can keep their faculties longer than the average Alzheimer's disease patient.

A vegan diet has also been shown to assist in reducing some symptoms of arthritis, such as reducing swelling in the joints, alleviating a significant amount of the pain associated with arthritis, and even helping with the general morning stiffness that those afflicted with arthritis feel in their joints upon waking.

Vegan Diet Cons

Possible Low Vegetable Intake

Ironically, though the vegan diet is meant to be all about plant-based foods, a lot of the time, vegetables don't actually play a large part in vegan diets, as a lot of people eat fruits, grains, beans, nuts, and seeds as well. There are also a lot of vegan processed foods, that due to additives and processing, may not be the best for an individual, which can even end up defeating the purpose of going vegan.

High Processed Food Intake

A lot of the time, vegan foods can be processed, such as tofurkey. Processed foods tend to include things such as sugars, oils, flour, and other additives, which make some vegan foods unhealthy. A lot of the calories in these processed foods come from these additives, as oatmeal, ice cream bars, tofurkey, frozen dinners, wheat thins, and other processed commercial foods can still be vegan, but unhealthy, and nearly totally devoid of proper nutrition.

Increasaed Need for Supplementation

However, as earlier stated, a vegan diet, to be properly balanced and to provide everything that a person needs to keep their body working properly and to stay healthy needs to be supplemented, due to the fact that while fruits, vegetables, and other plant matter is usually chock – full of nutrients, there are some micronutrients such as vitamin B 12 and calcium that is difficult and well – nigh impossible for people to obtain from a vegetable diet alone.

Constipation and Bloating

A lot of the time, those who eat vegan tend to have problems with gas, bloating, and being constipated. A lot of the foods that vegans eat, such as grains, beans, and nuts, include substances such as lectin and phytates that end up being difficult to digest, and wreaks havoc on our gut. These are protective substances for these plants, but make it very difficult to digest and absorb a lot of the time, which leads to these gastro intestinal problems.

Possible Poor Detoxification, Fatty Liver & Gallbladder Dysfunction

The problem with vegan diets is that they tend to be low in fat. Though fat has been demonized by a lot of popular culture, it is in fact necessary and in fact is quite good for you in certain quantities and according to certain types. Low fat diets end up making the body not need to use bile, which is a liquid that helps break down the fat. This excess bile ends up being stored in the gallbladder, and may thus end up forming gallstones and leading to difficulties in digestion. These gallstones are a known problem with those who adhere to vegan diets.

Paleo Diet Pros

The paleo diet presents a very balanced form of diet, allowing for protein, carbohydrate, and fat consumption in a good proportion. In addition to this, the paleo diet is built around whole foods, so much like veganism, it encourages using these in the diet, and these tend to be more sustainable.

The sustainability of the paleo diet should not be discounted, as this is important for ensuring the health of the environment. Simple foods are also usually sustainable, which makes for one's easy digestion, and still remains to be tasty and easily consumed.

Last but not least, the paleo diet is actually not very restrictive, and actually tends to cut out the worst offenders from the standard American diet, with a lot of paleo – friendly substitutes as needed. This means that a lot of the foods that are favorites of someone going on a paleo diet don't actually have to be cut out, but maybe simply modified a little bit.

Paleo Diet Cons

Low Veggie Intake

The paleo diet encourages simple, sustainable foods, but most people who adhere to the paleo diet tend to focus more on consuming proteins and fats, ignoring the aspect of eating their vegetables, only really giving it a token nod on their dinner plate, and not making it a priority.

Conventional Meat

A lot of the time, adherents of the paleo diet don't actually eat fully sustainable, and still eat conventional, farm raised meats. This means that a lot of the time, there are still antibiotics and hormones used in the farming of these animals that are used to put meat on the table. These hormones and antibiotics can end up negatively affecting one's body, and this can be detrimental to one's health, and reduce the effectiveness of the paleo diet. These antibiotics wreak havoc on a person's gut, with the microflora in the body being damaged, making it more difficult to digest things, and can lead to gut inflammation and increased disease risk.

Sweets and Treats

A lot of the time, a lot of paleo diet adherents still consume a large amount of sweets, thanks to the large market of paleo – compatible sweets. The high consumption of these sweets can still harm a person's diet, even if they're technically paleo compliant.

Processed Foods

Though paleo diet puts a large emphasis on natural foods, there are still a lot of packaged and processed foods in paleo friendly formats. As such, paleo bars, shakes, jerky, crackers, can all form a large part of a person's diet, even if they're technically on a paleo diet. These processed foods take away from the principles of a paleo diet, where whole foods are to be used in order to bring proper nutrients.

Digestion problems

Just because a food is healthy, doesn't mean that your body can properly handle it. A lot of the time, people who switch to the paleo diet have problems as their guts are not used to handling whole foods, or paleo compliant foods, even. A lot of the time, underlying gut problems make it difficult, as there can still be issues like leaky gut, parasitic infections, bacterial infections, or even simple food intolerances. This means that some people may not handle the paleo diet well, and thus the switch exacerbates their underlying problems.

Pegan Diet Balance

When it comes to fixing one's diet and nutrition, there really is no silver bullet or magic cure, and no one standard set of guidelines can really tell one what the best diet is for them, but the pegan diet philosophy seeks to balance everything as much as possible. It seeks to create a way of life, the true meaning of the word diet, coming from the latin *dieta*, rather than just a fad diet or a way to lose weight. Pegan diets actually stand for the way people used to eat, before people ended up creating fad diets and slapping labels onto everything. The ideas behind the pegan diet on emphasizing vegetables, eating other foods in moderation, reducing processed foods as much as possible – these tenets are all things that help improve one's health and dietary habits.

After all, pegan diets can be lumped into one real principle: eat real, proper food. Sure, snacks and sugary treats are still allowed, but in a very limited fashion. Thus, the principles of veganism and paleo diets are forwarded here, in improving sustainability, eating whole foods, and eating vegetables and non-processed foods, ignoring foods that are bad for you, or not as beneficial, and cutting out calorie dense foods with little to no nutritional value. Thus, the pegan diet is more flexible, and helps one operate with less rules, but thanks to the set principles, is still a great way to establish a healthier eating method.

WHAT CAN I EAT ON THE PEGAN DIET?

The pegan diet puts a large emphasis on eating whole foods, foods that have not been processed, or at least only have been processed to a limited degree before they reach one's dinner plate.

Vegetables

The primary food group of the pegan diet is vegetables. While a lot may have been excited by the fact that animal proteins and dairy are permissible, the main focus should still be vegetables. The standard pegan plate should be about seventy five percent greens. Most should be leafy greens, but low – glycemic fruits and other non starchy vegetables are also greatly emphasized in this diet, in order to help stabilize one's blood sugar. However, if there are no blood sugar problems, some starchy vegetables and sugary fruits can be introduced, but they should not take up too much space.

Responsibly Sourced Proteins

Though the pegan diet emphasizes vegetables, as earlier stated, animal proteins are also allowed, and in fact are still important in a diet that adheres to pegan principles. However, though proteins are important, remember that only 25% should be non-vegetables, and thus as there are other aspects, less than 25% of the plate should be made up of animal based proteins. These proteins should be responsibly sourced, preferably organic, pasture raised, and grass fed, avoiding conventionally farmed meats. Fish is also a great alternative to beef or poultry, provided that these fish are sustainably farmed or wild fish. Low mercury content fish such as sardines and wild salmon are encouraged.

Fats are key to maintaining proper health, as they allow us to be energetic and even provide nutritional benefits, but they should be sourced properly. Good fat sources would be most nuts, avoiding peanuts, seeds except for seed oils, as these tend to be heavily processed, avocados and olives, or their oils. Other good fat sources would be unrefined coconut oil, as well as fish, for their omega – 3 content, as fish oils are a great way to get omega 3s.

Whole Grains and Certain Legumes

Most grains are discouraged, as well as most legumes, though some are permissible. These whole grains and legumes should still be taken in limited quantities however, no more than half a cup, or about 125 grams of grains per meal, or one cup maximum of legume intake per day. The pegan – compatible grains would be black rice, quinoa, millet, amaranth, oats, and teff. The permissible legumes would be lentils, chickpeas, and pinto beans. Note however that if one needs to watch their blood sugar, grains and legumes are not recommended due to their high carbohydrate content.

WHAT SHOULD I AVOID?

The pegan diet is much more flexible than a paleo or a vegan diet, as most foods are allowed, but rather it is the quantity that tends to be restricted. However, some restrictions are still there, with some foods or even entire food groups being heavily discouraged. Some foods like dairy, while permitted, are to be used with caution, though foods made from sheep or goat milk are better than standard cow milk products. Legumes are also discouraged for the most part, as they wreak havoc on one's blood sugar, and for a lot of people, especially diabetics, this is something they have to keep watch over. Sugars are also permitted, but in very small quantities, and as a treat rather than a regular part of the diet. Refined oils as well as food additives are totally restricted, due to their heavy processing and their impact on one's body, causing inflammation, among others.

IS THE PEGAN DIET HEALTHY?

The quick answer: Yes. The long answer: the pegan diet helps improve one's health in many ways. One of the strongest points of the pegan diet is the greater emphasis it places on eating actual vegetables and fruits, which are some of the most nutrient dense and diverse foods people can eat. This incorporates a lot of fiber, vitamins, minerals, and plant compounds in one's diet. In addition, the pegan diet focuses on increasing healthy fats from fish, nuts, seeds, and other plants, which have a positive impact on one's health, especially on heart health. Furthermore, the emphasis on whole foods and sustainably sourced foods, and thus, the corresponding reduction in processed foods, helps improve overall diet quality.

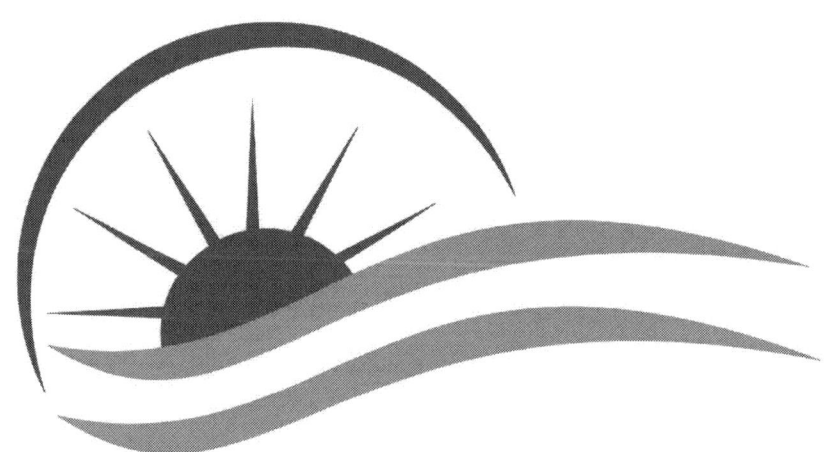

BREAKFAST RECIPES

Contents

Orange & Carrot Juice

Serves: 2 / Preparation time: 10 minutes

1 pound carrots, trimmed and scrubbed   4 oranges, peeled

- Add all ingredients into a juicer and extract the juice according to manufacturer's directions.
- Place the juice into glasses and serve immediately.

Per Serving: Calories: 266; Total Fat: 0.4g; Saturated Fat: 0.1g
Protein: 5.3g; Carbs: 65.6g; Fiber: 14.4g; Sugar: 40g

Green Fruit Juice

Serves: 2 / Preparation time: 10 minutes

2 medium green apples, cored and sliced

1 cup seedless green grapes

4 large kiwis, peeled and chopped

2 teaspoons fresh lime juice

- Add all ingredients into a juicer and extract the juice according to manufacturer's directions.
- Place the juice into glasses and serve immediately.

Per Serving: Calories: 261; Total Fat: 1.2g; Saturated Fat: 0g
Protein: 2.8g; Carbs: 66.6g; Fiber: 10.5g; Sugar: 48.4g

Apple Smoothie

Serves: 2 / Preparation time: 10 minutes

1 large granny smith apple, peeled, cored and chopped

1 large orange, peeled, seeded and sectioned

½ teaspoon lemon zest, grated freshly   ½ tablespoon fresh lemon juice

1½ cups chilled filtered water

- In a blender, place all the ingredients and pulse until smooth.
- Place the smoothie into glasses and serve immediately

Per Serving: Calories: 102; Total Fat: 0.3g; Saturated Fat: 0g
Protein: 1.2g; Carbs: 26.4g; Fiber: 5g; Sugar: 20.3g

Banana & Date Smoothie

Serves: 2 / Preparation time: 5 minutes

3-4 Medjool dates, pitted and chopped   2 large frozen bananas, peeled and sliced

1½ cups unsweetened chilled almond milk

- In a blender, place all the ingredients and pulse until smooth.
- Place the smoothie into glasses and serve immediately

Per Serving: Calories: 135; Total Fat: 3g; Saturated Fat: 0.4g
Protein: 2g; Carbs: 28.5g; Fiber: 3.8g; Sugar: 14.4g

Fruit & Greens Smoothie

Serves: 2 / Preparation time: 10 minutes

1 cup fresh baby spinach

1 cup fresh baby kale

1 frozen banana, peeled and chopped

½ cup frozen pineapple chunks

2 teaspoons chia seeds

1 tablespoon matcha green tea powder

1½ cups chilled unsweetened almond milk

- In a blender, place all the ingredients and pulse until smooth.
- Place the smoothie into glasses and serve immediately

Per Serving: Calories: 165; Total Fat: 3.8g; Saturated Fat: 0.4g
Protein: 3.6g; Carbs: 33.6g; Fiber: 4.6g; Sugar: 20.2g

Fruit Cocktail

Serves: 2 / Preparation time: 10 minutes

½ cup frozen mango, peeled, pitted and chopped

1 frozen banana, peeled and sliced

½ teaspoon organic vanilla extract

½ cup fresh orange juice

1 teaspoon fresh lemon juice

1 tablespoon coconut oil, melted

1 teaspoon maple syrup

3 tablespoons coconut yogurt

1 teaspoon fresh lime juice

¾ cup chilled filtered water

- In a high-speed blender, add all ingredients except coconut oil and pulse until smooth.
- While the motor is running, slowly, add coconut oil and pulse until creamy.
- Transfer into 2 large glasses and serve immediately.

Per Serving: Calories: 189; Total Fat: 7.6g; Saturated Fat: 6.2g
Protein: 1.6g; Carbs: 30.2g; Fiber: 2.4g; Sugar: 21g

Oats & Fruit Smoothie Bowl

Serves: 3 / Preparation time: 10 minutes

1 cup rolled oats, uncooked

2 ripe peaches, pitted and chopped

1 large orange, peeled, seeded and sectioned

1 large frozen banana, peeled and sliced

1 cup frozen mixed berries

1 tablespoon raw honey

1 cup unsweetened almond milk

1 cup mixed fruit

¼ cup raw pumpkin seeds, shelled

- In a high-speed blender, add all the ingredients except the fruit and pumpkin seeds and pulse until smooth.
- Transfer the mixture into 3 bowls evenly.
- Top with the mixed fruit and pumpkin seeds and serve.

Per Serving: Calories: 412; Total Fat: 9g; Saturated Fat: 1.5g
Protein: 10.2g; Carbs: 78g; Fiber: 10.8g; Sugar: 10.8g

Chia Seed Pudding

Serves: 2 / Preparation time: 10 minutes

1 cup unsweetened almond milk

¼ cup chia seeds

½ of small apple, cored and sliced

2 tablespoons maple syrup

¼ teaspoon organic vanilla extract

2 tablespoons almonds, chopped

- In a large bowl, add all ingredients except apple and almonds and stir to combine well.
- Cover and refrigerate for at least 30-40 minutes.
- Top with apple and almonds and serve.

Per Serving: Calories: 195; Total Fat: 9.9g; Saturated Fat: 0.8g
Protein: 4.9g; Carbs: 29.5g; Fiber: 7.6g; Sugar: 18g

Fruity Chia Seed Pudding

Serves: 4 / Preparation time: 10 minutes

2/3 cup unsweetened almond milk

½ of a frozen banana, peeled and sliced

½ cup chia seeds

2 cups frozen blueberries

5 large soft dates, pitted and chopped

- In a food processor, add all ingredients except chia seeds and pulse until smooth.
- Transfer the mixture into a bowl.
- Add chia seeds and stir to combine well.
- Refrigerate for 30 minutes, stirring after every 5 minutes.

Per Serving: Calories: 149; Total Fat: 5.9g; Saturated Fat: 0.5g
Protein: 4.1g; Carbs: 28g; Fiber: 8.1g; Sugar: 15.6g

Apple Porridge

Serves: 4 / Preparation time: 15 minutes / Cooking time: 5 minutes

2 cups unsweetened almond milk

2 large apples, peeled, cored and grated

3 tablespoons walnuts, chopped and divided

3 tablespoons pumpkin seeds, shelled

½ teaspoon organic vanilla extract

Pinch of ground cinnamon

½ small apple, cored and sliced

- In a large pan, add the milk, grated apple, 2 tablespoons of walnuts, pumpkin seeds, vanilla extract and cinnamon and mix well.
- Place the pan over medium-low heat and cook for about 3-4 minutes, stirring occasionally.
- Transfer the porridge into the serving bowls.
- Top with the remaining walnuts and apple slices and serve.

Per Serving: Calories: 165; Total Fat: 8.4g; Saturated Fat: 0.9g
Protein: 3.9g; Carbs: 22.1g; Fiber: 4.6g; Sugar: 14.7g

Banana Porridge

Serves: 6 / Preparation time: 15 minutes / Cooking time: 20 minutes

2 cups apple, peeled, cored and shredded

½ cup unsweetened coconut, shredded

1 teaspoon organic vanilla extract

½ cup cauliflower rice

1¾ cups unsweetened coconut milk

¾ cup fresh strawberries, hulled and sliced

- In a large pan, add all ingredients except strawberries over medium heat and bring to gentle simmer.
- Reduce the heat to low and simmer for about 15-20 minutes.
- Serve warm with the topping of strawberries.

Per Serving: Calories: 177; Total Fat: 12.1g; Saturated Fat: 10.7g
Protein: 1.6g; Carbs: 14.9g; Fiber: 3g; Sugar: 11g

Overnight Oatmeal

Serves: 3 / Preparation time: 10 minutes

1 cup rolled oats

2 bananas, peeled and mashed

1½ cups unsweetened coconut milk

2 tablespoons almonds, chopped

2 tablespoons chia seeds

2 teaspoons matcha green tea powder

Pinch of sea salt

- In a large bowl, add all ingredients except almonds and mix till well combined.
- Cover the bowl and refrigerate overnight.
- In the morning, remove from refrigerator.
- Top with almonds and serve.

Per Serving: Calories: 396; Total Fat: 22.2g; Saturated Fat: 15.7g
Protein: 7.8g; Carbs: 42g; Fiber: 7g; Sugar: 13.1g

Quinoa & Orange Porridge

Serves: 4 / Preparation time: 10 minutes / Cooking time: 20 minutes

2 cups water

1 cup dry red quinoa

½ cup unsweetened coconut milk

2 tablespoons maple syrup

¼ teaspoon fresh orange peel, grated finely

1 cup banana, peeled and sliced

- In a pan, mix together water and quinoa over medium heat and bring to boil.
- Reduce the heat to low and cook for about 10-15 minutes or until all liquid is absorbed, stirring occasionally.
- Stir in remaining ingredients and immediately, remove from heat.
- Top with banana slices serve.

Per Serving: Calories: 285; Total Fat: 9.9g; Saturated Fat: 6.7g
Protein: 7.1g; Carbs: 44.2g; Fiber: 4.6g; Sugar: 11.5g

Vanilla Crepes

Serves: 4 / Preparation time: 10 minutes / Cooking time: 8 minutes

2 tablespoons arrowroot powder

½ teaspoon ground cinnamon

4 organic eggs

1 tablespoon olive oil

2 tablespoons almond flour

Salt, as required

1 teaspoon organic vanilla extract

- In a bowl, add arrowroot powder, almond flour, cinnamon and salt and mix well.
- In another bowl, add the eggs and vanilla and beat until well combined.
- Add egg mixture into flour mixture and mix until well combined.
- In a non-stick frying pan, heat the oil over medium heat.
- Add desired sized mixture and swirl to coat the pan evenly in a thin layer
- Cook for about 1 minute per side.
- Repeat with the remaining mixture.

Per Serving: Calories: 137; Total Fat: 9.8g; Saturated Fat: 2g
Protein: 5.6g; Carbs: 5.3g; Fiber: 0.5g; Sugar: 0.6g

Egg White Waffles

Serves: 2 / Preparation time: 10 minutes / Cooking time: 8 minutes

¼ cup coconut flour

¼ cup unsweetened almond milk

1 tablespoon maple syrup

1 teaspoon organic baking powder

6 organic egg whites

Dash of organic vanilla extract

- Preheat the waffle iron and lightly grease it.
- In a large bowl, add the flour and baking powder and mix well.
- Add the remaining ingredients and mix until well combined.
- Place half of the mixture in preheated waffle iron.
- Cook for about 3-4 minutes or until waffles become golden brown.
- Repeat with the remaining mixture.
- Serve warm.

Per Serving: Calories: 156; Total Fat: 3.1g; Saturated Fat: 2g
Protein: 13.9g; Carbs: 17.9g; Fiber: 6.2g; Sugar: 7.7g

Blueberry Pancakes

Serves: 4 / Preparation time: 10 minutes / Cooking time: 20 minutes

½ cup coconut flour

2 drops liquid stevia

4 organic eggs

1 teaspoon organic vanilla extract

2 tablespoons olive oil

1 teaspoon baking soda

Pinch of salt

1 cup unsweetened almond milk

2 tablespoons fresh blueberries

2 tablespoons maple syrup

- In a large bowl, mix together the flour, baking soda and salt.
- In another bowl, add the egg, milk and vanilla extract and beat until well combined.
- Add the egg mixture into flour mixture and mix until well combined.
- Gently, fold in blueberries.
- In a large skillet, heat the oil over medium heat.
- Add desired amount of mixture and with the back of a wooden spoon, spread evenly.
- Cook for about 2-3 minutes.
- Carefully, flip the side and cook for about 1-2 minutes.
- Repeat with the remaining mixture.
- Serve warm with the drizzling of maple syrup.

Per Serving: Calories: 172; Total Fat: 12.5g; Saturated Fat: 2.7g
Protein: 6.1g; Carbs: 9.3g; Fiber: 1g; Sugar: 7g

Chicken & Zucchini Pancakes

Serves: 4 / Preparation time: 15 minutes / Cooking time: 40 minutes

4 cups zucchinis, shredded

¼ cup grass-fed cooked chicken, shredded

1 organic egg, beaten

Ground black pepper, as required

Salt, as required

¼ cup scallion, chopped finely

¼ cup coconut flour

2 tablespoons olive oil

- In a colander, add the zucchini and sprinkle with salt.
- Set aside for about 10-15 minutes.
- Then squeeze the zucchini well.
- In a bowl, add the zucchini and remaining ingredients and mix until we combined.
- In a large nonstick skillet, heat desired amount of oil over medium-low heat.
- Add ¼ cup of the zucchini mixture and with the back of a wooden spoon, spread evenly.
- Cook for 3-5 minutes per side.
- Repeat with the remaining mixture.
- Serve warm.

Per Serving: Calories: 113; Total Fat: 8.7g; Saturated Fat: 1.6g
Protein: 5.5g; Carbs: 4.9g; Fiber: 1.7g; Sugar: 2.2g

Pumpkin Muffins

Serves: 5 / Preparation time: 15 minutes / Cooking time: 25 minutes

1 cup almond flour

½ cup coconut flour

1 teaspoon baking soda

1 teaspoon pumpkin pie spice

Salt, as required

¼ cup raw honey

3 tablespoons coconut oil, melted

3 organic eggs

1 teaspoon organic vanilla extract

¾ cup homemade pumpkin puree

¼ cup pecans, chopped

- Preheat the oven to 325 degrees F. Grease 10 cups of a muffin pan.
- In a large bowl, mix together flours, baking soda and salt.
- In another bowl, add the remaining ingredients except pecans and beat until well combined.
- Add the egg mixture into flour mixture and mix until just combined.
- Fold in the pecans.
- Place the mixture into prepared muffin cups evenly.
- Bake for about 20-25 minutes or until a toothpick inserted in the center comes out clean.
- Remove from the oven and place the muffin pan onto a wire rack to cool for about 5 minutes.
- Carefully invert the muffins onto the wire rack to cool completely before serving.

Per Serving: Calories: 372; Total Fat: 27.8g; Saturated Fat: 9.4g
Protein: 4.7g; Carbs: 23.2g; Fiber: 4.8g; Sugar: 16.6g

Chicken & Veggie Muffins

Serves: 6 / Preparation time: 20 minutes / Cooking time: 40 minutes

8 large organic eggs, beaten
1 small red onion, chopped
1 teaspoon fresh rosemary, minced
1 pound grass-fed ground chicken
2 small carrots, peeled and grated
1 small red bell pepper, seeded and chopped
1 small green bell pepper, seeded and chopped
4 fresh mushrooms, chopped

2 tablespoons olive oil, divided
2 small garlic cloves, minced
¼ teaspoon red pepper flakes, crushed
Salt and ground black pepper, as required

- Preheat the oven to 355 degrees F. Lightly, grease a large 12 cups muffin pan.
- In a bowl, crack the eggs and beat well. Set aside.
- In a large skillet, heat 1 tablespoon of oil over medium heat and sauté the onion for about 5-6 minutes.
- Add the garlic, rosemary and red pepper flakes and sauté for about 1 minute.
- Add the chicken with a little salt and black pepper and cook for about 5-6 minutes.
- Transfer the chicken mixture into a bowl.
- In the same skillet, heat the remaining oil over medium heat and cook the carrot for about 2-3 minutes.
- Add the bell peppers and mushrooms and cook for about 1 minute.
- Stir in the salt and black pepper and cook for 2-3 minutes more.
- Transfer the vegetable mixture into the bowl with chicken mixture and mix until well combined.
- Add the beaten eggs and stir to combine well.
- Transfer the mixture into prepared muffin cups evenly.
- Bake for about 15-20 minutes or until top of muffins become golden brown.
- Remove from the oven and place the muffin pan onto a wire rack to cool for about 5 minutes.
- Carefully invert the muffins onto a platter and serve warm.

Per Serving: Calories: 308; Total Fat: 17.1g; Saturated Fat: 4.3g
Protein: 31.4g; Carbs: 7.1g; Fiber: 1.4g; Sugar: 4.1g

Zucchini Bread

Serves: 6 / Preparation time: 15 minutes / Cooking time: 45 minutes

½ cup coconut flour

Pinch of salt

2 teaspoons organic vanilla extract

1 cup zucchini, grated and squeezed

1½ teaspoons baking soda

¼ cup coconut oil, softened

1½ cups bananas, peeled and mashed

1 teaspoon orange zest, grated freshly

- Preheat the oven to 350 degrees F. Grease a loaf pan.
- In a large bowl, mix together the flour, baking soda and salt.
- In another bowl, add the coconut oil and vanilla extract and beat well.
- Add the banana and beat until well combined.
- Add the oil mixture into flour mixture and mix until just combined.
- Fold in zucchini and orange zest.
- Place the mixture into prepared loaf pan evenly.
- Bake for about 40-45 minutes or until a toothpick nested in the center comes out clean.
- Remove the loaf pan from oven and place onto a wire rack to cool for about 15-20 minutes.
- Carefully, remove the bread from the loaf pan and place onto the wire rack to cool completely before slicing.
- With a sharp knife, cut the bread loaf into desired sized slices and serve.

Per Serving: Calories: 124; Total Fat: 9.4g; Saturated Fat: 8.1g
Protein: 0.8g; Carbs: 10.1g; Fiber: 1.6g; Sugar: 5.2g

Banana Bread

Serves: 10 / Preparation time: 15 minutes / Cooking time: 1 hour

½ cup almond meal

¾ teaspoon baking soda

Pinch of salt

¼ cup maple syrup

2 teaspoons organic vanilla extract

½ cup coconut flour

1 teaspoon ground cinnamon

4 organic eggs

3½ tablespoons coconut oil, melted

2 medium bananas, peeled and mashed

- Preheat the oven to 340 degrees F. Grease a loaf pan.
- In a large bowl, mix together flours, baking soda, cinnamon and salt.
- In another bowl, add eggs, maple syrup, coconut oil and vanilla and beat until well combined.
- Add bananas and beat until well combined.
- Add the egg mixture into flour mixture and mix until just combined.
- Place the mixture into prepared loaf pan evenly.
- Bake for about 40-60 minutes or until a toothpick inserted in the center comes out clean.
- Remove bread from oven and let it cool slightly before slicing.
- Remove the loaf pan from oven and place onto a wire rack to cool for about 15-20 minutes.
- Carefully, remove the bread from the loaf pan and place onto the wire rack to cool completely before slicing.
- With a sharp knife, cut the bread loaf into desired sized slices and serve.

Per Serving: Calories: 146; Total Fat: 9.5g; Saturated Fat: 5g
Protein: 3.8g; Carbs: 12.7g; Fiber: 1.6g; Sugar: 8.1g

Caraway Seed Bread

Serves: 10 / Preparation time: 15 minutes / Cooking time: 35 minutes

1 1/3 cups almond flour

1 teaspoon organic baking powder

½ teaspoon onion powder

3 organic eggs

¼ cup water

¼ teaspoon white vinegar

1 tablespoon caraway seeds

½ teaspoon garlic powder

¼ teaspoon salt

¼ cup olive oil

1 tablespoon maple syrup

- Preheat oven to 350 degrees F. Line a loaf pan with parchment paper.
- In a large bowl, mix together almond flour, baking powder, caraway seeds, garlic powder, onion powder and salt.
- In another bowl, add the remaining ingredients and beat until well combined.
- Add the egg mixture into flour mixture and mix until just combined.
- Place the mixture into prepared loaf pan evenly.
- Bake for about 35 minutes or until a toothpick inserted in the center comes out clean.
- Remove the loaf pan from oven and place onto a wire rack to cool for about 15-20 minutes.
- Carefully, remove the bread from the loaf pan and place onto the wire rack to cool completely before slicing.
- With a sharp knife, cut the bread loaf into desired sized slices and serve.

Per Serving: Calories: 167; Total Fat: 14.5g; Saturated Fat: 1.7g
Protein: 1.8g; Carbs: 4.9g; Fiber: 1.9g; Sugar: 1.9g

Eggs in Avocado Cups

Serves: 4 / Preparation time: 10 minutes / Cooking time: 22 minutes

2 medium avocados, halved and pitted

6 cherry tomatoes, sliced

Salt and ground black pepper, as required

4 small organic eggs

¼ cup fresh basil leaves, chopped

- Preheat the oven to 450 degrees F. Lightly, grease a baking dish.
- Scoop out some flesh from each avocado half to create a cup.
- Arrange avocado halves into the prepared baking dish, cut side up.
- Carefully, crack each egg into each avocado half.
- Divide tomato slices over eggs evenly.
- Bake for about 20-22 minutes.
- Sprinkle with salt, and black pepper.
- Garnish with basil and serve.

Per Serving: Calories: 291; Total Fat: 123.7g; Saturated Fat: 5.3g
Protein: 8.2g; Carbs: 16.1g; Fiber: 9g; Sugar: 5.6g

Apple Omelet

Serves: 2 / Preparation time: 10 minutes / Cooking time: 10 minutes

4 teaspoons olive oil, divided

2 small green apples, cored and sliced thinly   ¼ teaspoon ground cinnamon

Pinch of ground cloves   Pinch of ground nutmeg

4 large organic eggs   ¼ teaspoon organic vanilla extract

Pinch of salt

- In a large nonstick frying pan, heat 1 teaspoon of oil over medium-low heat and cook the apple slices with spices for about 4-5 minutes, flipping once halfway through.
- Meanwhile, in a bowl, add the eggs, vanilla extract and salt and beat until fluffy.
- Add the remaining oil in the pan and let it heat.
- Place the egg mixture over apple slices evenly and cook for about 3-5 minutes or until desired doneness.
- Carefully, turn the pan over a serving plate and immediately, fold the omelet.
- Serve immediately.

Per Serving: Calories: 342; Total Fat: 19.8g; Saturated Fat: 4.5g
Protein: 13.2g; Carbs: 32g; Fiber: 5.6g; Sugar: 24.1g

Herbed Tomato Frittata

Serves: 6 / Preparation time: 15 minutes / Cooking time: 35 minutes

8 organic eggs, beaten

Salt and ground black pepper, as required

2 garlic cloves, minced

2 tablespoons fresh dill, chopped

1 teaspoon red pepper flakes, crushed

4 tomatoes, chopped

2 tablespoons fresh chives, chopped

- Preheat the oven to 325 degrees F. Grease a baking dish.
- In a large bowl, add eggs, salt and black pepper and beat well.
- Stir in tomatoes and herbs.
- Place the mixture into the prepared baking dish evenly.
- Bake for about 30-35 minutes.
- Remove from oven and set aside to cool for about 5-10 minutes before serving.

Per Serving: Calories: 104; Total Fat: 6.1g; Saturated Fat: 1.9g
Protein: 8.4g; Carbs: 4.8g; Fiber: 1.3g; Sugar: 2.7g

Chicken & Veggie Casserole

Serves: 6 / Preparation time: 20 minutes / Cooking time: 55 minutes

6 organic eggs

¼ teaspoon red pepper flakes, crushed

1 cup fresh kale, trimmed and chopped

1 cup fresh mushrooms, chopped

1 cup grass-fed cooked chicken, shredded

2 tablespoons fresh cilantro, minced

Salt and ground black pepper, as required

3 medium zucchinis, grated

1 medium onion, chopped

2 tablespoons almond flour

- Preheat the oven to 400 degrees F. Lightly, grease an 8x8-inch casserole dish.
- In a medium bowl, add eggs, cilantro, red pepper flakes, salt and black pepper and beat until well combined.
- In another large bowl, mix together all vegetables.
- Place the vegetable mixture into prepared casserole dish evenly and top with the shredded chicken, followed by
- Sprinkle with almond flour evenly.
- Top with egg mixture evenly.
- Bake for about 45-55 minutes or until top is golden brown.
- Remove from oven and set aside to cool for about 5-10 minutes before serving.

Per Serving: Calories: 144; Total Fat: 6.6g; Saturated Fat: 1.7g
Protein: 14.4g; Carbs: 7.4g; Fiber: 2g; Sugar: 3.1g

Veggies Quiche

Serves: 4 / Preparation time: 15 minutes / Cooking time: 20 minutes

6 organic eggs

½ cup unsweetened almond milk

Salt and ground black pepper, as required

1 cup fresh baby spinach, chopped

1 cup fresh baby kale, chopped

¼ cup fresh mushrooms, sliced

2 tablespoons red bell pepper, seeded and chopped

2 tablespoons green bell pepper, seeded and chopped

1 scallion, chopped

¼ cup fresh cilantro, chopped

1 tablespoon fresh chives, minced

- Preheat the oven to 400 degrees F. Lightly grease a pie dish.
- In a large bowl, add eggs, almond milk, salt and black pepper and beat well. Keep aside.
- In another bowl, add remaining ingredients.
- Place the veggie mixture in the bottom of prepared pie dish evenly and top with the egg mixture over vegetable mixture evenly.
- Bake for about 20 minutes or until a toothpick inserted in the center comes out clean.
- Remove from oven and set aside to cool for about 5-10 minutes before slicing before serving.

Per Serving: Calories: 114; Total Fat: 7.1g; Saturated Fat: 2.1g
Protein: 9.5g; Carbs: 3.7g; Fiber: 0.9g; Sugar: 1g

Zucchini with Eggs

Serves: 2 / Preparation time: 10 minutes / Cooking time: 5 minutes

1 tablespoon olive oil

2 large zucchinis, spiralized with blade C

2 organic eggs

2 small garlic clove, minced

Salt and ground black pepper, as required

- In a large skillet, heat the oil over medium heat and sauté the garlic for about 1 minute.
- Add the zucchini, salt and black pepper and cook for about 3-4 minutes.
- Transfer the zucchini mixture onto 2 large serving plates.
- Meanwhile, in a large pan, add 2-3-inches water over high heat and bring to a gentle simmer.
- Carefully, crack the eggs in water one by one.
- Cover the pan and turn off the heat.
- Place the pan covered for about 4 minutes or until desired doneness.
- Place the eggs over zucchini.
- Sprinkle the eggs with salt and black pepper and serve.

Per Serving: Calories: 179; Total Fat: 12g; Saturated Fat: 2.5g
Protein: 9.6g; Carbs: 12.2g; Fiber: 3.6g; Sugar: 6g

Sweet Potato & Bell Pepper Hash

Serves: 4/ Preparation time: 15 minutes / Cooking time: 32 minutes

1 tablespoon olive oil   1 medium onion, chopped

1 large sweet potato, peeled and cubed into ½-inch size

1 small green bell pepper, seeded and chopped

1 small red bell pepper, seeded and chopped

Salt and ground black pepper, as required   2 tablespoons water

¼ cup scallion (green part), chopped

- In a large skillet, heat oil over medium heat and sauté onion for about 4-5 minutes.
- Add the sweet potato and cook for about 4-5 minutes, stirring occasionally.
- Add the bell peppers and cook for about 1 minute.
- Add the salt, black pepper and water and stir to combine.
- Cover the skillet and cook for about 15-20 minutes, stirring occasionally.
- Stir in scallion and immediately remove from heat.
- Serve hot.

Per Serving: Calories: 96; Total Fat: 3.8g; Saturated Fat: 0.5g
Protein: 1.8g; Carbs: 15.3g; Fiber: 2.8g; Sugar: 6.8g

Quinoa & Coconut Granola

Serves: 4 / Preparation time: 15 minutes / Cooking time: 15 minutes

¾ cup uncooked red quinoa

½ cup coconut flakes

¼ cup almonds, chopped

¼ cup cashews, chopped

2 tablespoons raw pumpkin seeds, shelled

2 tablespoons chia seeds

½ teaspoon ground cinnamon

Pinch of ground ginger

Pinch of ground nutmeg

Pinch of ground cloves

Pinch of salt

3 tablespoons raw honey

2 tablespoons coconut oil, melted

½ cup raisins

1 medium banana, peeled and sliced

1 medium apple, cored and sliced

- Preheat the oven to 350 degrees F. Lightly grease a large baking sheet.
- In a large bowl, add quinoa, almonds, coconut flakes, both seeds, spices and salt and mix well.
- Add the honey and oil and stir until well combined.
- Transfer the quinoa mixture onto the prepared baking sheet and spread into an even layer.
- Bake for about 12-15 minutes, tossing occasionally.
- Remove from the oven and immediately, stir in the raisins.
- Set aside for about 10 minutes before serving.
- Serve with your choice of non-dairy milk and fruit's topping.

Per Serving: Calories: 492; Total Fat: 22.6g; Saturated Fat: 10.6g
Protein: 10.3g; Carbs: 70.4g; Fiber: 8.6g; Sugar: 34.4g

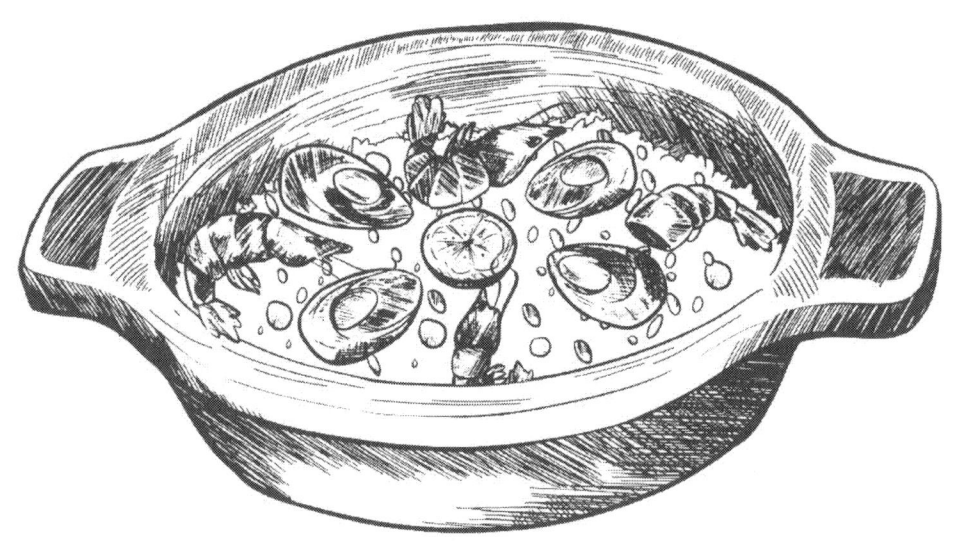

LUNCH RECIPES

Contents

Beet & Orange Salad

Serves: 3 / Preparation time: 15 minutes

2 oranges, peeled, seeded and sectioned

4 cups fresh arugula

2 tablespoon balsamic vinegar

2 beets, trimmed, peeled and sliced

3 tablespoons olive oil

Salt, as required

- In a large bowl, add all ingredients and gently, toss to coat.
- Serve immediately.

Per Serving: Calories: 216; Total Fat: 14.5g; Saturated Fat: 2.1g
Protein: 3g; Carbs: 22.1g; Fiber: 4.7g; Sugar: 17.4g

Broccoli & Carrot Salad

Serves: 2 / Preparation time: 15 minutes

1 small head broccoli with stem

2 medium carrots, peeled and spiralized with Blade C

¼ cup red onion, chopped

3 hard-boiled organic eggs, chopped

¼ cup fresh basil, chopped

1 garlic clove, minced

½ teaspoon lime zest, grated freshly

2 tablespoons extra-virgin olive oil

1 tablespoon fresh lime juice

Water, as required

Salt and ground black pepper, as required

2 tablespoons pumpkin seeds, roasted

- Cut the broccoli florets into bite-sized pieces.
- Spiralized the stem with Blade C.
- Transfer the chopped broccoli florets and spiralized stem into a large serving bowl.
- Add the carrot, onion and egg into the bowl with broccoli and mix.
- In a food processor, add remaining ingredients except pumpkin seeds and pulse until well combined.
- Pour mixture over vegetables and gently, toss to coat.
- Garnish with pumpkin seeds and serve.

Per Serving: Calories: 329; Total Fat: 24.9g; Saturated Fat: 8.6g
Protein: 14.1g; Carbs: 16.7g; Fiber: 4.9g; Sugar: 6g

Zoodles & Radish Salad

Serves: 4 / Preparation time: 15 minutes

2 tablespoons fresh lemon juice

2 teaspoons fresh lemon zest, grated

½ teaspoon Dijon mustard

½ teaspoon garlic powder

Salt and ground black pepper, as required

1/3 cup olive oil

3 medium zucchinis, spiralized with Blade C

1 bunch radishes, thinly sliced

- For dressing: in a small bowl, add the lemon juice, lemon zest, Dijon mustard, garlic powder, salt and black pepper and beat until well combined.
- Slowly, add the oil, beating continuously until well combined.
- In a large bowl, add the zucchini noodles, radishes and dressing and toss to coat well.
- 4. Serve immediately.

Per Serving: Calories: 178; Total Fat: 17.2g; Saturated Fat: 2.5g
Protein: 2.2g; Carbs: 6.9g; Fiber: 2.4g; Sugar: 3.6g

Greens Salad

Serves: 4/ Preparation time: 20 minutes / Cooking time: 6 minutes

1½ teaspoons fresh ginger, grated finely

3 tablespoons olive oil

3 teaspoons raw honey, divided

Salt, as required

2 tablespoons raw sunflower seeds

1 tablespoon raw sesame seeds

2 tablespoons apple cider vinegar

1 teaspoon sesame oil, toasted

½ teaspoon red pepper flakes, divided

1 tablespoon water

1 tablespoon raw pumpkin seeds, shelled

10 ounces mixed salad greens

- For dressing in a bowl, add the ginger, vinegar, both oils, 1 teaspoon of honey, ¼ teaspoon of the red pepper flakes and salt and beat until well combined.
- Set aside.
- In another bowl, add the remaining honey, remaining red pepper flakes and water and mix until well combined.
- Heat a medium nonstick skillet over medium heat and cook all the seeds for about 3 minutes, stirring continuously.
- Stir in the honey mixture and cook for about 3 minutes, stirring continuously.
- Transfer the seeds mixture onto a parchment paper and set aside to cool completely.
- Break the seeds mixture into small pieces.
- In a large bowl, add the greens, 2 teaspoons of the dressing and a little salt and toss to coat well.
- With your hands, rub the greens for about 30 seconds.
- Add the remaining dressing and seeds pieces and toss to coat well.
- Serve immediately.

Per Serving: Calories: 153; Total Fat: 14.6g; Saturated Fat: 2.1g
Protein: 2.2g; Carbs: 8.4g; Fiber: 0.6g; Sugar: 4.4g

Quinoa & Mango Salad

Serves: 2 / Preparation time: 15 minutes

1 large cucumber, spiralized with Blade C

½ cup cooked quinoa

3 tablespoons raw pumpkin seeds, shelled

1-2 fresh basil leaves, chopped

Salt and ground black pepper, as required

3 teaspoons extra-virgin olive oil

½ cup mango, peeled, pitted and cubed

¼ cup dried cranberries

½ teaspoon fresh ginger, grated

3 teaspoons balsamic vinegar

- In a large serving bowl, add all the ingredients and toss to coat well.
- Serve immediately.

Per Serving: Calories: 345; Total Fat: 15.9g; Saturated Fat: 2.5g
Protein: 10.6g; Carbs: 42.9g; Fiber: 5.5g; Sugar: 8.8g

Chilled Zucchini Soup

Serves: 4 / Preparation time: 15 minutes / Cooking time: 26 minutes

2 tablespoons extra-virgin coconut oil

2 small garlic cloves, minced

¼ teaspoon red pepper flakes, crushed

Salt and ground black pepper, as required

1½ cups water

1 small onion, chopped

1 teaspoon dried oregano, crushed

2 large zucchinis, chopped

2/3 cup homemade vegetable broth

1 small zucchini, spiralized with Blade C

- In a large pan, heat the oil over medium heat and sauté the onion for about 8- 9 minutes.
- Add the garlic, oregano and red pepper flakes and sauté for about 1 minute.
- Add the chopped zucchini, salt and black pepper and cook for about 8-10 minutes, stirring occasionally.
- Add the broth and water and bring to a boil over high heat.
- Reduce the heat to medium-low and simmer for about 10 minutes.
- Remove from the heat and set aside to cool slightly.
- In a blender, add the soup in batches and pulse until smooth.
- Transfer the soup into a large bowl and season with required salt and black pepper.
- Cover the bowl and refrigerate to chill.
- Top with spiralized zucchini and serve.

Per Serving: Calories: 112; Total Fat: 7.7g; Saturated Fat: 6.9g
Protein: 3.6g; Carbs: 9.3g; Fiber: 2.8g; Sugar: 4.4g

Egg Drop Soup

Serves: 6 / Preparation time: 10 minutes / Cooking time: 20 minutes

1 tablespoon olive oil

6 cups homemade chicken broth, divided

1 tablespoon arrowroot powder

Freshly ground white pepper, as required

1 tablespoon garlic, minced

2 organic eggs

1/3 cup fresh lemon juice

¼ cup scallion (green part), chopped

- In a large soup pan, heat oil over medium-high heat and sauté garlic for about 1 minute.
- Add 5½ cups of broth and bring to a boil over high heat.
- Reduce the heat to medium and simmer for about 5 minutes.
- Meanwhile, in a bowl, add eggs, arrowroot powder, lemon juice, white pepper and remaining broth and beat until well combined.
- Slowly, add egg mixture in the pan, stirring continuously.
- Simmer for about 5-6 minutes or until desired thickness of soup , stirring continuously
- Serve hot with the garnishing of scallion.

Per Serving: Calories: 92; Total Fat: 5.3g; Saturated Fat: 1.3g
Protein: 7g; Carbs: 3.4g; Fiber: 0.2g; Sugar: 1.2g

Broccoli Soup

Serves: 4 / Preparation time: 15 minutes / Cooking time: 35 minutes

1 tablespoon coconut oil

½ cup white onion, chopped

1 teaspoon ground turmeric

1 large head broccoli, cut into florets

1 bay leaf

Ground black pepper, as required

1 small avocado, peeled, pitted and chopped

1 celery stalk, chopped

Salt, as required

2 garlic cloves, minced

¼ teaspoon fresh ginger, grated

1/8 teaspoon cayenne pepper

5 cups homemade vegetable broth

1 tablespoon fresh lemon juice

- In a large soup pan, heat oil over medium heat and sauté celery, onion and some salt for about 3-4 minutes.
- Add turmeric and garlic and sauté for about 1 minute.
- Add desired mount of salt and remaining ingredients except avocado and lemon juice and bring to a boil
- Reduce the heat to medium-low and simmer, covered for about 25-30 minutes.
- Remove from heat and keep aside to cool slightly.
- In a blender, add soup and avocado in batches and pulse until smooth.
- Serve immediately with the drizzling of lemon juice.

Per Serving: Calories: 184; Total Fat: 13.5g; Saturated Fat: 5.1g
Protein: 3.1g; Carbs: 14.8g; Fiber: 6.9g; Sugar: 4.6g

Pumpkin Soup

Serves: 4 / Preparation time: 15 minutes / Cooking time: 25 minutes

2 teaspoons olive oil

1 onion, chopped

1 teaspoon fresh ginger, chopped

2 garlic cloves, chopped

2 tablespoons fresh cilantro, chopped

3 cups pumpkin, peeled, seeded and cubed

4¼ cups homemade vegetable broth

Salt and ground black pepper, as required

¾ cup coconut cream

2 tablespoons fresh lime juice

- In a large soup pan, heat the oil over medium heat and sauté the onion, ginger, garlic and cilantro for about 4-5 minutes.
- Add the pumpkin and broth and bring to a boil
- Reduce the heat to low and simmer, covered for about 15 minutes.
- Remove from the heat and set aside to cool slightly.
- Transfer the mixture into a high-speed blender in batches with ½ cup of the coconut cream and pulse until smooth.
- Return the soup into the pan over medium heat and cook for about 3-5 minutes or until heated through.
- Serve hot with the topping of the remaining coconut cream.

Per Serving: Calories: 216; Total Fat: 13.6g; Saturated Fat: 10.1g
Protein: 3.5g; Carbs: 23.8g; Fiber: 8g; Sugar: 10.9g

Meatballs with Apple Chutney

Serves: 6 / Preparation time: 20 minutes / Cooking time: 20 minutes

For Meatballs

1 pound ground turkey

1 tablespoon olive oil

1 teaspoon dehydrated onion flakes, crushed

½ teaspoon granulated garlic

½ teaspoon ground cumin

½ teaspoon red pepper flakes, crushed

Salt, as required

For Chutney

3 medium tart apples, peeled, cored and chopped

½ handful of golden raisins

3 tablespoons maple syrup

2 tablespoons almond butter

1 tablespoon apple cider vinegar

¼ cup water

¼ teaspoon ground cumin

Pinch of red pepper flakes, crushed

Salt, as required

- Preheat the oven to 400 degrees F. Line a large baking sheet with parchment paper.
- For meatballs in a large mixing bowl, add all ingredients and mix until well combined.
- Make equal-sized balls from the mixture.
- Arrange the meatballs onto prepared baking sheet in a single layer.
- Bake for about 15-20 minutes or until done completely.
- Meanwhile, for chutney in a medium pan, mix together all ingredients over medium-high heat.
- Cover the pan and cook for about 6-8 minutes, stirring occasionally.
- Uncover and cook for 2-3 minutes or until desired thickness.
- Remove from heat and let it cool slightly.
- With a potato masher, mash the apple pieces slightly to form a chunky mixture forms.
- Serve meatballs with chutney.

Per Serving: Calories: 306; Total Fat: 14g; Saturated Fat: 1.9g
Protein: 22.4g; Carbs: 28.5g; Fiber: 3.6g; Sugar: 21.6g

Black Beans Meatballs

Serves: 8 / Preparation time: 20 minutes / Cooking time: 19 minutes

1 pound ground turkey breast

1 cup cooked black beans, mashed roughly

1 small yellow bell pepper, seeded and chopped finely

1 small green bell pepper, seeded and chopped finely

½ cup fresh parsley, chopped

¼ cup olive oil

Salt and ground black pepper, as required

4 cups cherry tomatoes, halved

- For meatballs: in a large bowl, add all ingredients and mix until well combined.
- Make equal-sized balls from the mixture.
- In a skillet, heat oil over medium heat and cook the meatballs for about 5-7 minutes or until golden brown from all sides.
- Cover the skillet and cook for about 5 minutes more.
- Divide the cherry tomatoes and meatballs onto serving plates and serve.

Per Serving: Calories: 271; Total Fat: 11.1g; Saturated Fat: 2.2g
Protein: 22.7g; Carbs: 21.1g; Fiber: 5.3g; Sugar: 4.4g

Veggie Meatballs

Serves: 6 / Preparation time: 15 minutes / Cooking time: 30 minutes

½ cup carrot, peeled and grated

½ cup yellow squash, grated

1 pound grass-fed ground beef

¼ of a small onion, chopped finely

8 cups lettuce, torn

½ cup zucchini, grated

Salt, as required

1 organic egg, beaten

1 garlic clove, minced

- Preheat the oven to 400 degrees F. Line a large baking sheet with parchment paper.
- Set a large colander over the sink.
- In the sink, place the carrot, zucchini and yellow squash and sprinkle with 2 pinches of salt.
- Set aside for at least 10 minutes.
- Transfer the veggies onto a paper towel and squeeze out all the moisture of veggies.
- In a large bowl, add the squeezed vegetables, beef, egg, onion, garlic, herbs and desired amount of salt and mix until well combined.
- Make equal-sized balls from the mixture.
- Arrange the meatballs onto prepared baking sheet in a single layer.
- Bake for about 25-30 minutes or until done completely.
- Divide the lettuce and meatballs onto serving plates and serve.

Per Serving: Calories: 163; Total Fat: 8.3g; Saturated Fat: 3.3g
Protein: 17g; Carbs: 4.2g; Fiber: 1g; Sugar: 1.7g

Oats & Black Beans Burgers

Serves: 6 / Preparation time: 20 minutes / Cooking time: 40 minutes

½ cup rolled oats

¼ cup raw pumpkin seeds, shelled

2 (15-ounce) cans black beans, rinsed, drained and divided

2 cups carrots, peeled and grated

½ teaspoon ground coriander

½ teaspoon ground cumin

½ teaspoon red pepper flakes, crushed

¼ teaspoon cayenne pepper

¼ teaspoon onion powder

¼ teaspoon garlic powder

Salt and ground black pepper, as required

1 tablespoon olive oil

8 cups fresh baby greens

- Preheat the oven to 300 degrees F. Line a large baking sheet with parchment paper.
- In a food processor, add the pumpkin seeds and oats and pulse until chopped roughly.
- Add ¾ of the beans, carrots, spices and oil and pulse until well combined.
- Transfer the mixture into a large bowl.
- Fold in remaining beans.
- With your wet hands, make 6 equal-sized patties from the mixture.
- Arrange the patties onto the prepared baking sheet in a single layer.
- Bake for about 20 minutes per side.
- Divide the greens onto serving plates.
- Top each with 1 burger and serve.

Per Serving: Calories: 227; Total Fat: 6.6g; Saturated Fat: 0.9g
Protein: 11.4g; Carbs: 31.4g; Fiber: 9.3g; Sugar: 2.5g

Salmon & Quinoa Burgers

Serves: 6 / Preparation time: 20 minutes / Cooking time: 20 minutes

2 tablespoons ground flax seeds

1 cooked large beet, peeled and chopped

½ cup cooked quinoa

½ cup fresh parsley, chopped

Salt and ground black pepper, as required

5 tablespoons hot water

2 (6-ounce) cans salmon

½ cup fresh kale, chopped

2 garlic cloves, peeled

8 cups fresh baby spinach

- Preheat the oven to 350 degrees F. Line a baking sheet with parchment paper.
- In a bowl, add the flaxseeds and water and mix well.
- In a food processor, add the beet and pulse until chopped.
- Add the flax seeds mixture and remaining ingredients a chucky mixture is formed.
- With your wet hands, make 6 equal-sized patties from the mixture.
- Arrange the patties onto the prepared baking sheet in a single layer.
- Bake for about 15-20 minutes, flipping once halfway through.
- Divide the spinach onto serving plates.
- Top each with 1 burger and serve.

Per Serving: Calories: 162; Total Fat: 5.3g; Saturated Fat: 0.7g
Protein: 15.2g; Carbs: 14.1g; Fiber: 3.1g; Sugar: 1.6g

Beef & Veggie Burgers

Serves: 4 / Preparation time: 15 minutes / Cooking time: 8 minutes

1 pound grass-fed ground beef

1 medium raw beetroot, trimmed, peeled and chopped finely

1 carrot, peeled and chopped finely

1 small brown onion, chopped finely

1 tablespoon fresh rosemary, chopped finely

Salt and ground black pepper, as required

2-3 tablespoons coconut oil

6 cups salad greens

- In a large mixing bowl, add all ingredients except oil and mix until well combined.
- Make 12 equal-sized patties from mixture.
- In a large skillet, heat the oil over medium heat and cook the patties for about 3-4 minutes per side or until golden brown.
- Divide the greens onto serving plates.
- Top each with 1 burger and serve.

Per Serving: Calories: 198; Total Fat: 12g; Saturated Fat: 7g
Protein: 16.4g; Carbs: 5.6g; Fiber: 1.6g; Sugar: 2.3g

Turkey & Apple Burgers

Serves: 4 / Preparation time: 15 minutes / Cooking time: 12 minutes

12 ounces lean ground turkey

½ of apple, peeled, cored and grated

½ of red bell pepper, chopped finely

¼ cup red onion, minced

2 small garlic cloves, minced

1 tablespoon fresh ginger, minced

2½ tablespoons fresh cilantro, chopped

2 tablespoons curry paste

1 teaspoon ground cumin

1 teaspoon olive oil

6 cups fresh baby spinach

- Preheat the grill to medium heat. Grease the grill grate.
- For burgers: in a large bowl, add all ingredients and mix until well combined.
- Make 4 equal-sized burgers from mixture. Brush the burgers with olive oil evenly.
- Grill the burgers for about 5-6 minutes per side.
- Divide the spinach onto serving plates.
- Top each with 1 burger and serve.

Per Serving: Calories: 223; Total Fat: 12.1g; Saturated Fat: 2.1g
Protein: 19g; Carbs: 11.1g; Fiber: 2.3g; Sugar: 4.2g

Veggies Burgers

Serves: 4 / Preparation time: 15 minutes / Cooking time: 40minutes

1 large organic egg

½ teaspoon red pepper flakes, crushed

¼ cup coconut oil, melted

1 large zucchini, spiralized with Blade C and chopped

1 large sweet potato, peeled, spiralized with Blade C and chopped

2 tablespoons fresh cilantro leaves, chopped

¼ teaspoon ground cumin

Salt and ground black pepper, as required

2 tablespoons almond flour

6 cups lettuce, torn

- Preheat the oven to 375 degrees F. Line 2 baking sheets with greased parchment papers.
- In a large bowl, add the egg and spices and beat well.
- Add the butter and flour and mix until well combined.
- Add the remaining ingredients and mix until well combined.
- Make equal sized patties from the mixture.
- Arrange the patties onto prepared baking sheets in a single layer.
- Bake for about 10 minutes.
- Now, reduce the temperature of oven to 350 degrees F.
- Bake for about 15 minutes.
- Carefully, flip the side of patties and bake for about 15 minutes.
- Divide the lettuce onto serving plates.
- Top each with 1 burger and serve.

Per Serving: Calories: 217; Total Fat: 17.2g; Saturated Fat: 12.3g
Protein: 3.8g; Carbs: 13.9g; Fiber: 3.1g; Sugar: 4.9g

Turkey & Beans Lettuce Wraps

Serves: 2 / Preparation time: 15 minutes / Cooking time: 13 minutes

4 ounces lean ground turkey

2 tablespoons sugar-free tomato sauce

1/8 teaspoon ground cumin

Salt and ground black pepper, as required

1 cup tomato, chopped

4 tablespoons avocado, peeled, pitted and chopped

¼ cup onion, minced

1/8 teaspoon garlic powder

2 teaspoons extra-virgin olive oil

1/3 cup cooked black beans

4 large lettuce leaves

- In a bowl, add turkey, onion, tomato sauce and spices and mix until well combined.
- In a large skillet, heat the oil over medium heat and cook the turkey mixture for about 8-10 minutes.
- Add the beans and tomato and stir to combine.
- Reduce the heat to low and cook for about 2-3 minutes.
- Remove from the heat and set aside to cool.
- Arrange the lettuce leaves onto serving plates.
- Divide turkey mixture onto each lettuce leaf and top with avocado pieces.
- Serve immediately.

Per Serving: Calories: 297; Total Fat: 13g; Saturated Fat: 2.8g
Protein: 19.7g; Carbs: 27.9g; Fiber: 7.8g; Sugar: 4.6g

Shrimp Lettuce Wraps

Serves: 6 / Preparation time: 20 minutes / Cooking time: 4 minutes

For Salsa

1 mango, peeled, pitted and chopped   ¼ cup red onion, chopped finely

½ cup red bell pepper, seeded and chopped finely

¼ cup fresh cilantro, chopped   1 jalapeño pepper, chopped finely

2 tablespoons fresh lime juice   Salt and ground black pepper, as required

For Wraps

1 teaspoon olive oil

2 pounds large shrimp, peeled, deveined and chopped

½ teaspoon ground cumin   1 tablespoon red chili powder

Salt and ground black pepper, as required   12 lettuce leaves

- For salsa: in a large bowl, add all the ingredients and gently, stir to combine.
- Set aside until using.
- In a large skillet, heat the oil over medium heat and cook the shrimp with spices for about 3-4 minutes.
- Remove from the heat and set aside to cool slightly.
- Arrange the lettuce leaves onto serving plates.
- Divide the shrimp mixture onto each lettuce leaf and top with mango salsa.
- Serve immediately.

Per Serving: Calories: 170; Total Fat: 1g; Saturated Fat: 0.2g
Protein: 29.1g; Carbs: 12.8g; Fiber: 1.3g; Sugar: 8.5g

Chicken & Pineapple Kabobs

Serves: 6 / Preparation time: 15 minutes / Cooking time: 22 minutes

For Sauce

3 cups pineapple, chopped

¼ cup coconut aminos

2 tablespoons cashew butter

1 tablespoon maple syrup

1 tablespoon fresh lime juice

½ teaspoon red pepper flakes, crushed

¼ teaspoon garlic powder

¼ teaspoon onion powder

Salt and ground black pepper, as required

For Kabobs

2 pounds grass-fed skinless, boneless chicken thighs, cubed

2 cups fresh pineapple, cubed

- For sauce: in a food processor, add all the ingredients and pulse until smooth.
- Transfer the sauce into a pan over medium heat and cook for about 10-12 minutes, stirring occasionally.
- Remove from the heat and set aside.
- Preheat the grill to medium-high heat. Grease the grill grate.
- Thread the chicken and pineapple cubes onto the metal skewers.
- Place the skewers onto the grill and cook for about 8-10 minutes, flipping after every 2-3 minutes.
- In the last 2 minutes of cooking, coat the kabobs with sauce evenly.
- Serve with remaining sauce as a dipping sauce.

Per Serving: Calories: 309; Total Fat: 8.2g; Saturated Fat: 2.6g
Protein: 35.5g; Carbs: 24g; Fiber: 2.1g; Sugar: 15.6g

Chicken & Veggie Kabobs

Serves: 4 / Preparation time: 15 minutes / Cooking time: 8 minutes

1 teaspoon paprika

½ teaspoon ground coriander

Pinch of ground ginger

Salt and ground black pepper, as required

½ tablespoon extra-virgin olive oil

1 pound grass-fed boneless, skinless chicken breast, cubed

1 large green bell pepper, seeded and cut into 1-inch pieces

12 cherry tomatoes, halved

¼ teaspoon cayenne pepper

1 teaspoon ground cumin

Pinch of ground cumin

2 teaspoons fresh lemon juice

1 medium red onion, cut into 1-inch pieces

- Preheat the oven to 425 degrees F. Lightly, grease a large baking sheet.
- For marinade: in a large bowl, mix together spices, lemon juice and oil.
- Add chicken cubes and coat with marinade generously.
- Cover and refrigerate for about 20 minutes.
- Remove chicken from marinade and thread onto skewers with bell pepper, tomato and onion.
- Place the skewers in prepared baking sheet in a single layer.
- Bake for about 10 minutes or until desired doneness.
- Serve warm.

Per Serving: Calories: 176; Total Fat: 5g; Saturated Fat: 0.3g
Protein: 25.2g; Carbs: 6.8g; Fiber: 1.7g; Sugar: 3.7g

Veggie Kabobs

Serves: 4 / Preparation time: 15 minutes / Cooking time: 10 minutes

For Marinade

2 garlic cloves, chopped

1 teaspoon fresh oregano

½ teaspoon cayenne pepper

¼ cup olive oil

2 tablespoons fresh ginger, chopped

1 teaspoon fresh basil

Salt and ground black pepper, as required

For Veggies

½ head of cauliflower, cut into large florets

4 large button mushrooms, quartered

1 medium red bell pepper, seeded and cut into large cubes

1 medium onion, cut into large cubes

1 large zucchinis, cut into thick slices

Salt and ground black pepper, as required

- For marinade: in a food processor, add all the ingredients and pulse until well combined.
- In a large bowl, add all the vegetables.
- Pour marinade mixture over vegetables and toss to coat well.
- Cover and refrigerate to marinate for at least 6-8 hours.
- Preheat the grill to medium-high heat. Grease the grill grate.
- Remove vegetables from marinade and thread onto pre-soaked wooden skewers.
- Place the skewers onto the grill and cook for about 8-10 minutes or until done completely, flipping occasionally.
- Serve warm.

Per Serving: Calories: 168; Total Fat: 13.2g; Saturated Fat: 1.9g
Protein: 3.4g; Carbs: 12.9g; Fiber: 3.5g; Sugar: 5.4g

Shrimp Kabobs

Serves: 4 / Preparation time: 15 minutes / Cooking time: 8 minutes

1 jalapeño pepper, chopped

1 (1-inch) fresh ginger, minced

1 cup unsweetened coconut milk

1½ pounds medium shrimp, peeled and deveined

1 large garlic clove, chopped

1/3 cup fresh mint leaves

¼ cup fresh lime juice

- In a food processor, add jalapeño, garlic, ginger, mint, coconut milk, lime juice and fish sauce and pulse until smooth.
- Add the shrimp and coat with marinade generously.
- Cover and refrigerate to marinate for at least 1-2 hours.
- Preheat the grill to medium-high heat. Grease the grill grate.
- Remove shrimp from marinade and thread onto pre-soaked wooden skewers with avocado and watermelon.
- Grill, turning once for about 6-8 minutes or until done completely.
- Serve warm.

Per Serving: Calories: 307; Total Fat: 16.4g; Saturated Fat: 12.7g
Protein: 38.2g; Carbs: 4.6g; Fiber: 2g; Sugar: 2.1g

Shrimp & Watermelon Kabobs

Serves: 4 / Preparation time: 15 minutes / Cooking time: 4 minutes

1/3 cup plus 1 tablespoon olive oil, divided

1/3 cup fresh mint leaves, chopped

2 garlic cloves, minced

½ teaspoon red pepper flakes

1 pound jumbo shrimp, peeled and deveined

3 cups seedless watermelon, peeled and cubed into 1-inch size

3 tablespoons fresh lime juice

1 tablespoon fresh thyme leaves

2-3 teaspoons lime zest, grated

Salt and ground black pepper, as required

- In a small bowl, add 1/3 cup of oil, lime juice, 1/3 cup of mint, thyme, garlic, lime zest, red pepper flakes, salt and black pepper and beat until well combined.
- In a large bowl, add the shrimp and half of the marinade and toss to coat well.
- Cover the bowl and refrigerate for about 1 hour.
- Reserve remaining marinade in refrigerator until using.
- Preheat the grill to high heat. Grease the grill grate.
- Thread the watermelon onto metal skewers and coat with the remaining oil.
- Place the skewers onto the grill and cook for about 1-2 minutes, flipping occasionally.
- Coat the shrimp with some of the reserved marinade and thread onto skewers.
- Place the skewers onto the grill and cook for about 1 minute per side.
- Arrange the watermelon and shrimp onto a platter.
- Drizzle with the remaining marinade and serve.

Per Serving: Calories: 335; Total Fat: 24.8g; Saturated Fat: 3.6g
Protein: 21.4g; Carbs: 10.5g; Fiber: 1.4g; Sugar: 9.1g

Spinach in Creamy Sauce

Serves: 4 / Preparation time: 10 minutes / Cooking time: 15 minutes

2 tablespoons coconut oil

1 garlic clove, minced

1 small head cauliflower, chopped roughly

1 tablespoon fresh lemon zest, grated

1/8 teaspoon ground cinnamon

2 pounds fresh spinach, chopped roughly

1 small onion, chopped

Salt and ground black pepper, as required

1 cup homemade vegetable broth

1 tablespoon Dijon mustard

1 cup unsweetened coconut milk

- In a large skillet, melt the coconut oil over medium heat and sauté the onion and garlic for about 2 minutes.
- Add the cauliflower and cook for about 1-2 minutes.
- Stir in the broth and bring to a boil.
- Reduce the heat to low and simmer, covered for about 5-7 minutes.
- Remove from heat and stir in remaining ingredients except spinach.
- With an immense blender, blend the spinach until a smooth puree forms.
- Meanwhile, in a large microwave-safe bowl, add spinach and cook on high for about 4 minutes.
- Remove from microwave and set aside to cool completely.
- Then squeeze the spinach completely.
- Add spinach in creamy sauce and stir to combine.
- Serve immediately.

Per Serving: Calories: 287; Total Fat: 22.6g; Saturated Fat: 18.8g
Protein: 10.8g; Carbs: 17.8g; Fiber: 8.6g; Sugar: 5.6g

Broccoli with Kale

Serves: 6 / Preparation time: 15 minutes / Cooking time: 20 minutes

2 tablespoons olive oil

2 garlic cloves, minced

1 cup fresh kale, tough ribs removed and chopped

1 head broccoli, cut into florets

1 teaspoon ground cumin

Salt, as required

1 onion, chopped

2 cups cherry tomatoes, halved

1 teaspoon red chili powder

- In a large skillet, heat the oil over medium heat and sauté onion for about 4-5 minutes.
- Add garlic and sauté for about 1 minute.
- Add the kale, broccoli florets, tomatoes, cumin, chipotle powder and salt and cook for about 10 minutes, stirring occasionally.
- Serve warm.

Per Serving: Calories: 82; Total Fat: 5.1g; Saturated Fat: 0.7g
Protein: 2.4g; Carbs: 8.8g; Fiber: 2.6 g; Sugar: 3.1g

Cabbage with Apple

Serves: 4 / Preparation time: 15 minutes / Cooking time: 12 minutes

2 teaspoons coconut oil

1 onion, sliced thinly

1 tablespoon fresh thyme, chopped

1 tablespoon apple cider vinegar

1 large apple, cored and sliced thinly

1½ pounds cabbage, chopped finely

1 fresh red chili, chopped

- In a nonstick skillet, melt 1 teaspoon of coconut oil over medium heat and stir fry apple for about 2-3 minutes.
- Transfer the apple into a bowl.
- In the same skillet, melt 1 teaspoon of coconut oil over medium heat and sauté onion for about 2-3 minutes.
- Add cabbage and stir fry for about 4-5 minutes.
- Add apple, thyme and vinegar and cook, covered for about 1 minute.
- Serve warm.

Per Serving: Calories: 105; Total Fat: 2.6g; Saturated Fat: 2g
Protein: 2.7g; Carbs: 20.7g; Fiber: 6.5g; Sugar: 12.5g

Kale with Cranberries

Serves: 4 / Preparation time: 15 minutes / Cooking time: 5 minutes

1 tablespoon extra-virgin olive oil

1 large shallot, sliced thinly

12-16 fresh kale leaves, trimmed and torn

2 tablespoons dried unsweetened cranberries

2 tablespoons fresh orange juice

2 tablespoons pumpkin seeds, toasted

1 small garlic cloves, chopped

1 teaspoon fresh orange zest, grated

2 tablespoons water

½ tablespoon balsamic vinegar

Salt and ground black pepper, as required

¼ cup pine nuts

- In a large skillet, heat the oil over medium heat and sauté the garlic and shallots for about 2 minutes.
- Add the orange zest, kale and water and cook for about 2-3 minutes.
- Stir in the cranberries, vinegar and orange juice and cook, covered for about 1-2 minutes.
- Uncover the skillet and cook for about 1-2 minutes or until all the liquid is absorbed.
- Remove from the heat and stir in the salt and black pepper.
- Stir in the pumpkin seeds and pine nuts and serve.

Per Serving: Calories: 191; Total Fat: 11.3g; Saturated Fat: 1.3g
Protein: 6.7g; Carbs: 19g; Fiber: 2.8g; Sugar: 1.2g

Sweet & Sour Shrimp

Serves: 3 / Preparation time: 15 minutes / Cooking time: 10 minutes

For Sauce

3 tablespoons fresh orange juice

1 tablespoon coconut aminos

For Shrimp

¾ pound shrimp, peeled and deveined

1 tablespoon extra-virgin olive oil

1 teaspoon fresh ginger, minced

1 tablespoon raw honey

½ tablespoon balsamic vinegar

½ tablespoons arrowroot powder

2 garlic cloves, minced

- For sauce: in a bowl, all ingredients and mix well. Keep aside.
- In another bowl, add shrimp and arrowroot powder and toss to coat well.
- In a large skillet, heat oil over medium-high heat and sauté garlic and ginger for about 1 minute
- Add shrimp and cook for about 3 minutes.
- Add sauce and cook for about 2 minutes, stirring continuously.
- With a slotted spoon, transfer the shrimp into a bowl.
- Cook for about 2-4 minutes or until desired thickness, stirring continuously.
- Serve shrimp with the topping of sauce.

Per Serving: Calories: 219; Total Fat: 6.7g; Saturated Fat: 1.3g
Protein: 26.1g; Carbs: 12.5g; Fiber: 0.2g; Sugar: 7.1g

Quinoa with Green Peas

Serves: 4 / Preparation time: 15 minutes / Cooking time: 15 minutes

2 cups plus 1 tablespoon water, divided

Salt, as required

¼ cup fresh basil, chopped finely

2 tablespoons olive oil

1 teaspoon maple syrup

1 cup dry quinoa, rinsed

1 cup fresh green peas, shelled

2 tablespoons fresh lemon juice

2 teaspoons Dijon mustard

Ground black pepper, as required

- In a pan, add 2 cups of the water, quinoa and a pinch of salt over medium-high heat and bring to a boil.
- Reduce the heat to low and simmer, partially covered for about 15 minutes or until all the liquid is absorbed.
- Meanwhile, in a microwave-safe dish, add the peas and remaining water.
- Cover the bowl and microwave on high for about 3-4 minutes.
- Stir the peas and microwave for about 3-5 minutes more.
- Remove from the microwave and drain any liquid from the dish.
- Remove the pan of the quinoa from the heat and set aside, covered for about 5 minutes.
- Uncover the pan and with a fork, fluff the quinoa.
- In a large bowl, add the quinoa, peas and basil and mix.
- In another bowl, add the lemon juice, oil, maple syrup, mustard, salt and black pepper and beat until well combined.
- Pour the oil mixture over the quinoa mixture and toss to coat well.
- Serve warm.

Per Serving: Calories: 254; Total Fat: 9.9g; Saturated Fat: 1.4g
Protein: 8.2g; Carbs: 34g; Fiber: 5g; Sugar: 3.2g

DINNER RECIPES

Contents

Chicken Salad

Serves: 8 / Preparation time: 15 minutes

For Dressing

½ teaspoon fresh ginger, minced   ¼ cup fresh lemon juice

2 tablespoons Dijon mustard   2 tablespoons olive oil

Salt and ground black pepper, as required

For Salad

3 cups grass-fed cooked chicken, shredded

½ of small pineapple, peeled, cored and sliced thinly

4 plum tomatoes, thinly sliced lengthwise   1½ pounds Napa cabbage, shredded

½ cup scallions, sliced thinly

- For dressing: in a bowl, add all the ingredients and beat until well combined.
- For salad: in a large serving bowl, add all the ingredients and mix.
- Place the vinaigrette over salad and gently toss to coat well.
- Serve immediately.

Per Serving: Calories: 153; Total Fat: 5.7g; Saturated Fat: 1.1g
Protein: 17.5g; Carbs: 9.2g; Fiber: 2.4g; Sugar: 6g

Beef & Plum Salad

Serves: 4 / Preparation time: 15 minutes / Cooking time: 10 minutes

4 teaspoons fresh lemon juice, divided

1½ tablespoons extra-virgin olive oil, divided

1 pound grass-fed flank steak, trimmed

1 teaspoon raw honey

3 plums, pitted and sliced thinly

Salt and ground black pepper, as required

Cooking spray, as required

8 cups fresh baby arugula

- In a large bowl, place 1 teaspoon of lemon juice, 1½ teaspoons of oil, salt and black pepper and mix well.
- Add the steak and coat with mixture generously.
- Grease a nonstick skillet with a little cooking spray and heat over medium-high heat.
- Add the beef steak and cook for about 5-6 minutes per side.
- Transfer the steak onto a cutting board and set aside for about 10 minutes before slicing.
- With a sharp knife, cut the beef steak diagonally across grain in desired size slices.
- In a large bowl, add the remaining lemon juice, oil, honey, sea salt and black pepper and beat well.
- Add the arugula and toss well.
- Divide arugula onto 4 serving plates.
- Top with beef slices and plum slices evenly and serve.

Per Serving: Calories: 304; Total Fat: 15.1g; Saturated Fat: 4.7g
Protein: 33g; Carbs: 9g; Fiber: 1.3g; Sugar: 7.6g

Salmon & Veggie Salad

Serves: 2 / Preparation time: 15minutes

6 ounces grilled salmon, cut into bite-sized pieces

1 medium zucchini, spiralized with Blade C

1 medium cucumber, peeled and spiralized with Blade C

½ cup celery stalk, chopped   ½ cup unsweetened coconut milk

1 small garlic clove, minced   Salt and ground black pepper, as required

2 organic hard-boiled large eggs, peeled and chopped

- In a large serving bowl, mix together salmon, zucchini, cucumber and celery.
- In another bowl, add the coconut milk, garlic and seasoning and mix until well combined.
- Pour the coconut milk mixture over vegetables and gently, toss to coat.
- Top with chopped eggs and serve.

Per Serving: Calories: 367; Total Fat: 24.9g; Saturated Fat: 15.1g
Protein: 26.6g; Carbs: 13.7g; Fiber: 3.6g; Sugar: 7g

Chicken & Zucchini Soup

Serves: 4 / Preparation time: 15 minutes / Cooking time: 20 minutes

1 tablespoon olive oil

½ cup onion, chopped

1 cup carrot, peeled and chopped

2 garlic cloves, minced

2 tablespoons fresh rosemary, chopped

4½ cups homemade chicken broth

1¼ cups fresh spinach, torn

1¼ cups grass-fed cooked chicken, shredded

1¼ cups zucchini, spiralized with Blade C

Salt and ground black pepper, as required

2 tablespoons fresh lemon juice

- In a large soup pan, heat the oil over medium heat and sauté the onion and carrots for about 8-9 minutes.
- Add the garlic and rosemary and sauté for about 1 minute.
- Add the broth and spinach and bring to a boil over high heat.
- Reduce the heat to medium-low and simmer for about 5 minutes.
- Add the cooked chicken and zucchini and simmer for about 5 minutes.
- Stir in the salt, black pepper and lemon juice and remove from heat.
- Serve hot.

Per Serving: Calories: 174; Total Fat: 6.8g; Saturated Fat: 1.5g
Protein: 19.5g; Carbs: 8.3g; Fiber: 2.4g; Sugar: 3.6g

Quinoa Soup

Serves: 6 / Preparation time: 15 minutes / Cooking time: 35 minutes

1 tablespoon coconut oil	3 carrots, peeled and chopped
3 celery stalks, chopped	1 onion, chopped
4 garlic cloves, minced	4 cups tomatoes, chopped
1 cup red lentils, rinsed and drained	½ cup dried quinoa, rinsed and drained
1½ teaspoons ground cumin	1 teaspoon red chili powder
5 cups homemade vegetable broth	2 cups fresh spinach, chopped

- In a large pan, heat the oil over medium heat and sauté the celery, onion and carrot for about 8 minutes.
- Add the garlic and sauté for about 1 minute.
- Add the remaining ingredients except spinach and bring to a boil.
- Reduce the heat to low and simmer, covered for about 20 minutes.
- Stir in spinach and simmer for about 3-4 minutes.
- Serve hot.

Per Serving: Calories: 268; Total Fat: 5.1g; Saturated Fat: 2.5g
Protein: 16.4g; Carbs: 40.2g; Fiber: 13.9g; Sugar: 6.9g

Beef & Veggie Stew

Serves: 5 / Preparation time: 15 minutes / Cooking time: 2 hours 5 minutes

1 pound grass-fed beef stew meat, trimmed and cubed

Salt and ground black pepper, as required

2 medium carrots, peeled and chopped

1 medium onion, chopped

3 cups fresh tomatoes, chopped finely

1 cup frozen peas, thawed

2 tablespoons olive oil, divided

2 celery stalks, chopped

1 cup pumpkin, peeled and cube

4 cups homemade beef broth

¼ cup fresh cilantro, chopped

- Season the beef with a little salt and black pepper evenly.
- In a large heavy-bottomed pan, heat 1 tablespoon of oil over medium heat and sear beef for about 4-5 minutes.
- Transfer the beef into a large bowl and keep aside.
- In the same pan, heat remaining oil over medium heat and sauté carrot, celery and onion for about 5 minutes.
- Add the pumpkin and tomatoes and sauté for about 5 minutes.
- Add the broth and beef and bring to a boil over high heat.
- Reduce the heat to low and simmer, covered for about 1 hour.
- Uncover and simmer for about 35 minutes.
- Stir in the peas, salt and black pepper and simmer for 15 minutes more.
- Serve hot with the garnishing of cilantro.

Per Serving: Calories: 328; Total Fat: 12.8g; Saturated Fat: 3.4g
Protein: 35.1g; Carbs: 18.1g; Fiber: 5.7g; Sugar: 8.7g

Chicken Chili

Serves: 6 / Preparation time: 15 minutes / Cooking time: 40 minutes

4 cups homemade chicken broth, divided

3 cups cooked black beans, divided

1 tablespoon extra-virgin olive oil

1 large onion, chopped

2 medium poblano peppers, seeded and chopped

1 jalapeño pepper, seeded and chopped

4 garlic cloves, minced

1 teaspoon dried thyme, crushed

1½ tablespoons ground coriander

1 tablespoon ground cumin

½ tablespoon ancho chili powder

4 cups grass-fed cooked chicken, shredded

1 tablespoon fresh lime juice

¼ cup fresh cilantro, chopped

- In a food processor, add 1 cup of broth and 1½ cups of black beans and pulse until smooth.
- Transfer the beans puree into a bowl and set aside.
- In a large pan, heat the oil over medium heat and sauté the onion, poblano and jalapeño for about 4-5 minutes.
- Add the garlic, spices and sea salt and sauté for about 1 minute.
- Add the beans puree and remaining broth and bring to a boil.
- Reduce the heat to low and simmer for about 20 minutes.
- Stir in the remaining beans, chicken and lime juice and bring to a boil.
- Reduce the heat to low and simmer for about 5-10 minutes.
- Serve hot with the topping of cilantro.

Per Serving: Calories: 321; Total Fat: 7.4g; Saturated Fat: 1.4g
Protein: 38.3g; Carbs: 23.7g; Fiber: 7g; Sugar: 2.4g

Beef Chili

Serves: 8 / Preparation time: 15 minutes / Cooking time: 2¼ hours

2 tablespoons extra-virgin olive oil

1 large onion, chopped

1 large green bell pepper, seeded and chopped

4 garlic cloves, minced

1 jalapeño pepper, chopped

1 teaspoon dried thyme, crushed

1 teaspoon dried basil, crushed

2 tablespoons red chili powder

1 tablespoon ground cumin

1 teaspoon ground allspice

2 pounds grass-fed lean ground beef

3 cups fresh tomatoes, chopped finely

2 cups homemade chicken broth

1 cup water

- In a large pan, heat the oil over medium heat and sauté the onion and bell pepper for about 5-7 minutes.
- Add garlic, jalapeño pepper, herbs, spices and black pepper and sauté for about 1 minute.
- Add the beef and cook for about 4-5 minutes.
- Stir in the tomatoes and cook for about 2 minutes.
- Add the broth and water and bring to a boil.
- Reduce the heat to low and simmer, covered for about 2 hours.
- Serve hot.

Per Serving: Calories: 277; Total Fat: 14.6g; Saturated Fat: 5.2g
Protein: 25.7g; Carbs: 8g; Fiber: 2.3g; Sugar: 3.7g

Lamb Chili

Serves: 6 / Preparation time: 15 minutes / Cooking time: 2 hours

1½ tablespoons extra-virgin olive oil, divided

1 cup onion, chopped   6 large garlic cloves, minced

2 dried New Mexico chiles, stemmed, seeded and torn

3 dried ancho chiles, stemmed, seeded and torn

2 teaspoons dried oregano, crushed   1½ teaspoons ground cumin

2 large plum tomatoes, chopped   2 cups homemade chicken broth

1 pound grass-fed lamb stew meat, trimmed and cubed

Salt and ground black pepper, as required   15 ounces cooked kidney beans

- In an oven-proof pan, heat 1 tablespoon of oil over medium heat and sauté the onion for about 4-5 minutes.
- Add the garlic, both chiles and spices and sauté for about 1 minute.
- Add the tomatoes and broth and bring to a boil.
- Reduce the heat to medium-low and simmer, covered for about 30 minutes.
- Preheat the oven to 325 degrees F. Arrange a rack in the center of the oven.
- Remove the pan from heat and set aside to cool slightly.
- Transfer the chile mixture into a blender and pulse until pureed.
- Return the puree in the same pan.
- Meanwhile, in another pan, heat the remaining oil over medium-high heat and cook the lamb with salt and black pepper k for about 3-4 minutes.
- Transfer the cooked lamb in the pan with puree and stir to combine.
- Cover the pan and bake for about 50 minutes.
- Remove pan from the oven and place over medium-low heat.
- Simmer, uncovered for about 25 minutes.
- Stir in kidney beans and simmer for about 5 minutes.
- Serve hot.

Per Serving: Calories: 430; Total Fat: 8.3g; Saturated Fat: 2.4g
Protein: 40g; Carbs: 49.7g; Fiber: 12.4g; Sugar: 4.4g

Glazed Chicken Thighs

Serves: 6 / Preparation time: 10 minutes / Cooking time: 20 minutes

3 garlic cloves, minced

½ cup fresh orange juice

1 tablespoon apple cider vinegar

2 tablespoons coconut aminos

½ teaspoon orange blossom water

¼ teaspoon ground ginger

¼ teaspoon ground cinnamon

Salt, as required

2 pounds grass-fed skinless, bone-in chicken thighs

- For marinade: in a large bowl, place all ingredients except chicken and mix well.
- Add the chicken and coat with marinade generously.
- Cover the bowl of chicken and refrigerate for about 2 hours.
- Remove the chicken from bowl, reserving marinade.
- Heat a large nonstick wok, over medium-high heat and cook the chicken for about 5-6 minutes or until golden brown.
- Flip the side and cook for about 4 minutes.
- Add the reserved marinade and bring to a boil.
- Now, reduce the heat to medium-low heat and cook, covered for about 6-8 minutes or until sauce becomes thick.
- Serve hot.

Per Serving: Calories: 305; Total Fat: 11.3g; Saturated Fat: 3.1g
Protein: 44g; Carbs: 8.3g; Fiber: 0.1g; Sugar: 1.8g

Grilled Chicken Breast

Serves: 4 / Preparation time: 15 minutes / Cooking time: 20 minutes

1 (1-inch) piece fresh ginger, minced

2 garlic cloves, minced

1 cup fresh pineapple juice

¼ cup coconut aminos

¼ cup extra-virgin olive oil

1 teaspoon ground cinnamon

1 teaspoon ground cumin

Salt, as required

4 grass-fed skinless, boneless chicken breasts

- In a large Ziploc bag add all ingredients and seal it.
- Shake the bag to coat the chicken with marinade well.
- Refrigerate to marinade for about 1 hour.
- Preheat the grill to medium-high heat. Grease the grill grate.
- Place the chicken breasts onto the grill and cook for about 10 minutes per side.
- Serve hot.

Per Serving: Calories: 341; Total Fat: 17.9g; Saturated Fat: 3.7g
Protein: 32.1g; Carbs: 12.6g; Fiber: 0.6g; Sugar: 6.3g

Chicken with Pineapple & Bell Peppers

Serves: 5 / Preparation time: 20 minutes / Cooking time: 25 minutes

1 tablespoon extra-virgin olive oil

1 large onion, chopped

1 garlic clove, minced

1 teaspoon fresh ginger, minced

2 grass-fed skinless, boneless chicken breasts, cubed

2 cups fresh pineapple, cubed

2 tomatoes, seeded and chopped

1 medium red bell pepper, seeded and chopped

1 medium green bell pepper, seeded and chopped

1 medium orange bell pepper, seeded and chopped

2 tablespoons coconut aminos

1 tablespoon apple cider vinegar

Ground black pepper, as required

- In a large skillet, heat oil over medium heat.
- Add onion and sauté for about 4-5 minutes.
- Add garlic and ginger and sauté for about 1 minute.
- Add chicken and cook for about 10 minutes or until browned from all sides.
- Add pineapple, tomatoes and bell peppers and cook for about 5-6 minutes or until vegetables become tender.
- Add the coconut aminos, vinegar and pepper and cook for about 2-3 minutes.
- Serve hot.

Per Serving: Calories: 194; Total Fat: 5.6g; Saturated Fat: 1.3g
Protein: 17.1g; Carbs: 20.5g; Fiber: 3.2g; Sugar: 12.2g

Chicken with Fruit & Veggies

Serves: 3 / Preparation time: 15 minutes / Cooking time: 15 minutes

2 zucchinis, spiralized with Blade C
1½ teaspoons olive oil
¾ cup rhubarb, chopped
10 ounces grass-fed skinless, boneless chicken breasts, cubed
4 teaspoons raw honey
¼ cup plus 2 teaspoons fresh orange juice, divided
1 tablespoon fresh lime juice
½ cup fresh strawberries, hulled and sliced
2 tablespoons almonds, toasted and slivered

Salt, as required
½ teaspoon fresh ginger, minced

1 teaspoon fresh lime zest, grated finely

2 teaspoons fresh mint leaves, minced

- Arrange a large strainer over the sink.
- Place the zucchini noodles in a strainer and sprinkle with a pinch of salt.
- Set aside to release the excess moisture.
- In a large skillet, heat the oil over medium heat and cook the ginger and rhubarb for about 2-3 minutes.
- Stir in the chicken cubes and cook for about 4-5 minutes.
- Add the honey, lime zest, ¼ cup of orange juice, lime juice and a pinch of salt and stir to combine.
- Now, increase the heat to high and bring to a boil.
- Now, reduce the heat to medium and simmer for about 4-5 minutes, stirring occasionally.
- Remove from the heat.
- Meanwhile, squeeze the moisture from zucchini and pat dry with paper towels.
- In a small bowl, place the remaining orange juice and mint and mix.
- Divide the zucchini noodles in serving plates and drizzle with mint mixture.
- Place the chicken mixture, strawberries and almonds over zucchini noodles and gently stir to combine.
- Serve immediately.

Per Serving: Calories: 236; Total Fat: 8.1g; Saturated Fat: 1.8g
Protein: 24.2g; Carbs: 18.8g; Fiber: 3.2g; Sugar: 13.4g

Chicken & Broccoli Casserole

Serves: 6 / Preparation time: 15 minutes / Cooking time: 45 minutes

6 (6-ounce) grass-fed skinless, boneless chicken thighs

3 broccoli heads, cut into florets

4 garlic cloves, minced

¼ cup extra-virgin olive oil

1 teaspoon dried oregano, crushed

1 teaspoon dried rosemary, crushed

Salt and ground black pepper, as required

- Preheat the oven to 375 degrees F. Grease a large baking dish.
- In a large bowl, add all ingredients and toss to coat well.
- In the bottom of prepared baking dish, arrange the broccoli florets and top with chicken breasts in a single layer.
- Bake for about 45 minutes.
- Serve hot.

Per Serving: Calories: 329; Total Fat: 14.9g; Saturated Fat: 3.5g
Protein: 41.5g; Carbs: 8.8g; Fiber: 3.3g; Sugar: 2g

Stuffed Turkey Breast

Serves: 12 / Preparation time: 20 minutes / Cooking time: 2 hours

For Turkey Rub
1 (5-pound) whole, bone-in turkey breast
2 tablespoons fresh thyme leaves, chopped   2 tablespoons fresh rosemary, chopped
2 tablespoons olive oil
For Stuffing
1 small onion, thinly sliced   1 apple, peeled and thinly sliced
1 pear, peeled and thinly sliced   ¼ cup dried cranberries
For Glaze
2 cups fresh apple juice, divided   1 tablespoon olive oil
1 tablespoon brown mustard   ½ tablespoon coconut sugar

- Preheat the oven to 325 degrees F. Arrange a rack in a roasting pan.
- Arrange turkey breast into the prepared roasting pan, skin-side up.
- With your fingers, gently loosen the skin from the meat, making deep pockets between the skin and meat.
- For rub: in a small bowl, mix together fresh herbs and oil.
- Rub half of herb mixture on the meat and then, spread the remaining paste evenly over the top of the skin.
- For stuffing: in a bowl, mix together all ingredients.
- Stuff each pocket with the stuffing mixture.
- In the bottom of roasting pan, pour 1 cup of apple juice.
- Roast for about 1¾-2 hours. (If skin becomes brown during roasting, then cover the pan with a piece of foil).
- Meanwhile, for glaze: in a pan, add remaining apple juice, oil, mustard and brown sugar and bring to a boil.
- Reduce the heat and simmer until thick glaze is formed.
- In the last 30 minutes of cooking, coat turkey breast with glaze evenly.
- Remove from oven and cut turkey into desired slices before serving.

Per Serving: Calories: 290; Total Fat: 9.2g; Saturated Fat: 1.5g
Protein: 32.5g; Carbs: 19.1g; Fiber: 2.4g; Sugar: 14.5g

Glazed Flank Steak

Serves: 4 / Preparation time: 15 minutes / Cooking time: 12 minutes

2 tablespoons arrowroot flour
1 pound grass-fed flank steak, cut into ¼-inch thick slices
½ cup plus 1 tablespoon coconut oil, divided
1 teaspoon ground ginger
1/3 cup raw honey
½ cup coconut aminos

Salt and ground black pepper, as required

2 garlic cloves, minced
Pinch of red pepper flakes, crushed
½ cup homemade beef broth
3 scallions, chopped

- In a bowl, add the arrowroot flour, salt and black pepper and mix well.
- Coat the beef slices with arrowroot flour mixture evenly.
- Shake off the excess arrowroot flour mixture and set aside for about 10-15 minutes.
- For sauce: in a pan, melt 1 tablespoon of coconut oil over medium heat and sauté the garlic, ginger powder and red pepper flakes for about 1 minute.
- Add the honey, broth and coconut aminos and stir to combine well.
- Now, increase the heat to high and cook for about 3 minutes, stirring continuously.
- Remove from the heat and set aside.
- In a large skillet, melt the remaining coconut oil over medium heat and stir fry the beef for about 2-3 minutes.
- Remove the oil from skillet and stir fry for about 1 minute.
- Stir in the honey sauce and cook for about 3 minutes.
- Stir in the scallion and cook for about 1 minute more.
- Serve hot.

Per Serving: Calories: 586; Total Fat: 36.9g; Saturated Fat: 27.5g
Protein: 32.8g; Carbs: 31.6g; Fiber: 0.5g; Sugar: 23.6g

Beef with Cauliflower

Serves: 4 / Preparation time: 15 minutes / Cooking time: 12 minutes

1 tablespoon coconut oil

4 garlic cloves, minced

1 pound grass-fed beef sirloin steak, cut into bite-sized pieces

3½ cups cauliflower florets

3 tablespoons coconut aminos

¼ cup fresh cilantro leaves, chopped

- In a large skillet, heat the oil over medium heat and sauté the garlic for about 1 minute.
- Add beef and stir to combine.
- Increase the heat to medium-high and cook for about 6-8 minutes or until browned from all sides.
- Meanwhile, in a pan of boiling filtered water, add cauliflower and cook for about 5-6 minutes.
- Drain the cauliflower completely.
- Add the cauliflower and coconut aminos in skillet with beef and cook for about 2-3 minutes.
- Serve with the garnishing of cilantro.

Per Serving: Calories: 278; Total Fat: 10.6g; Saturated Fat: 5.6g
Protein: 36.3g; Carbs: 7.9g; Fiber: 2.3g; Sugar: 2.1g

Beef with Lentils

Serves: 6 / Preparation time: 15 minutes / Cooking time: 50 minutes

3 tablespoons extra-virgin olive oil, divided   1 onion, chopped

1 tablespoon fresh ginger, minced   4 garlic cloves, minced

3 plum tomatoes, chopped finely

2 cups dried red lentils, soaked for 30 minutes and drained

2 cups homemade chicken broth   2 teaspoons cumin seeds

½ teaspoon cayenne pepper   1 pound grass-fed lean ground beef

1 jalapeño pepper, seeded and chopped   2 scallions, chopped

- In a Dutch oven, heat 1 tablespoon of oil over medium heat and sauté the onion, ginger and garlic for about 5 minutes.
- Stir in the tomatoes, lentils and broth and bring to a boil
- Reduce the heat to medium-low and simmer, covered for about 30 minutes.
- Meanwhile, in a skillet, heat remaining oil over medium heat.
- Add the cumin seeds and sauté for about 30 seconds.
- Add the paprika and sauté for about 30 seconds.
- Transfer the mixture into a small bowl and set aside.
- In the same skillet, add the beef and cook for about 4-5 minutes.
- Add jalapeño and scallion and cook for about 4-5 minutes.
- Add the spiced oil mixture and stir to combine well.
- Transfer the beef mixture into the simmering lentils and simmer for about 10-15 minutes or until desired doneness.
- Serve hot.

Per Serving: Calories: 469; Total Fat: 13,3g; Saturated Fat: 3.1g
Protein: 42.3g; Carbs: 45.1g; Fiber: 21.1g; Sugar: 4.2g

Ground Beef with Peas

Serves: 6 / Preparation time: 15 minutes / Cooking time: 40 minutes

2 tablespoons olive oil

1 large onion, chopped finely

½ tablespoon fresh ginger, minced

1 teaspoon ground cumin

2 medium tomatoes, seeded and chopped

Salt and ground black pepper, as required

2 tablespoons fresh cilantro, chopped

1 pound grass-fed lean ground beef

2 garlic cloves, minced

1 teaspoon ground coriander

¼ teaspoon chili powder

½ cup homemade chicken broth

2¼ cups fresh peas, shelled

- In a large skillet, heat the oil over medium heat and cook the beef for about 4-5 minutes or until browned completely.
- With a slotted spoon, transfer the beef into a large bowl.
- In the same skillet, add onion and sauté for about 4-6 minutes.
- Add the garlic, ginger, coriander, cumin and chili powder and sauté for about 1 minute.
- Add the tomatoes and cook for about 2-3 minutes, crushing completely with the back of spoon.
- Stir in the beef and broth and bring to a boil.
- Reduce the heat to medium-low and simmer, covered for about 8-10 minutes, stirring occasionally.
- Stir in peas and cook for 10-15 minutes.
- Remove from heat and serve hot with the garnishing of almonds and cilantro leaves.

Per Serving: Calories: 243; Total Fat: 11.9g; Saturated Fat: 3.8g
Protein: 19.5g; Carbs: 12.7g; Fiber: 4g; Sugar: 5.3g

Stuffed Bell Peppers

Serves: 5 / Preparation time: 20 minutes / Cooking time: 40 minutes

5 large bell peppers, tops and seeds removed

1 tablespoon coconut oil

½ large onion, chopped

½ teaspoon dried oregano

½ teaspoon dried thyme

Salt and ground black pepper, as required

1 pound grass-fed ground beef

1 large zucchini, chopped

3 tablespoons homemade tomato paste

- Preheat the oven to 350 degrees F. Grease a small baking dish.
- In a large pan of the boiling water, place the bell peppers and cook for about 4-5 minutes.
- Remove from the water and place onto a paper towel, cut side down.
- Meanwhile, in a large nonstick skillet, melt coconut oil over medium heat and sauté onion for about 3-4 minutes.
- Add the ground beef, oregano, salt, and pepper and cook for about 8-10 minutes.
- Add zucchini and cook for about 2-3 minutes.
- Remove from the heat and drain any juices from the beef mixture.
- Add the tomato paste and stir to combine.
- Arrange the bell peppers into the prepared baking dish, cut side upward.
- Stuff the bell peppers with the beef mixture evenly and bake for 15 minutes.
- Serve warm.

Per Serving: Calories: 247; Total Fat: 12.1g; Saturated Fat: 6g
Protein: 21.1g; Carbs: 14.5g; Fiber: 3.1g; Sugar: 8.9g

Broiled Lamb Shoulder

Serves: 6 / Preparation time: 10 minutes / Cooking time: 10 minutes

2 tablespoons fresh ginger, minced

2 tablespoons garlic, minced

¼ cup fresh lemongrass stalk, minced

¼ cup fresh orange juice

¼ cup coconut aminos

Ground black pepper, as required

2 pounds grass-fed lamb shoulder, trimmed

- In a bowl, add all ingredients except lamb shoulder and mix well.
- In a baking dish, place the lamb shoulder and coat the lamb with half of the marinade mixture generously.
- Reserve remaining mixture.
- Refrigerate to marinate overnight.
- Preheat the broiler of oven. Place a rack in a broiler pan and arrange about 4-5-inches from the heating element.
- Remove lamb shoulder from refrigerator and shake off excess marinade.
- Broil for about 4-5 minutes per side.
- Serve alongside the reserved marinade as a sauce.

Per Serving: Calories: 306; Total Fat: 11.2g; Saturated Fat: 4g
Protein: 42.9g; Carbs: 5.3g; Fiber: 0.3g; Sugar: 1g

Pan Seared Lamb Chops

Serves: 4 / Preparation time: 15 minutes / Cooking time: 6 minutes

4 garlic cloves, peeled

Salt, as required

1 teaspoon black mustard seeds, crushed finely

2 teaspoons ground cumin

1 teaspoon ground ginger

1 teaspoon ground coriander

½ teaspoon ground cinnamon

Ground black pepper, as required

1 tablespoon coconut oil

8 grass-fed medium lamb chops, trimmed

- Place the garlic cloves onto a cutting board and sprinkle with some salt.
- With a knife, crush the garlic until a paste forms.
- In a bowl, mix together garlic paste and spices.
- With a sharp knife, make 3-4 cuts on both side of the chops.
- Rub the chops with garlic mixture generously.
- In a large skillet, melt the coconut oil over medium heat and cook the chops for about 2-3 minutes per side or until desired doneness.
- Serve hot.

Per Serving: Calories: 571; Total Fat: 24.7g; Saturated Fat: 10.4g
Protein: 80.3g; Carbs: 2.3g; Fiber: 0.5g; Sugar: 0.1g

Poached Salmon

Serves: 3 / Preparation time: 15 minutes / Cooking time: 12 minutes

3 garlic cloves, crushed

1/3 cup fresh orange juice

3 (6-ounce) salmon fillets

1½ teaspoons fresh ginger, grated finely

3 tablespoons coconut aminos

- In a bowl, add all the ingredients except salmon and mix well.
- In the bottom of a large pan, place the salmon fillet.
- Place the ginger mixture over the salmon and set aside for about 15 minutes.
- Place the pan over high heat and bring to a boil.
- Reduce the heat to low and simmer, covered for about 10-12 minutes or until desired doneness.
- Serve hot.

Per Serving: Calories: 260; Total Fat: 10.6g; Saturated Fat: 1.5g
Protein: 33.5g; Carbs: 7.5g; Fiber: 0.2g; Sugar: 2.4g

Shrimp with Zoodles

Serves: 4 / Preparation time: 15 minutes / Cooking time: 8 minutes

2 tablespoons coconut oil

1 pound shrimp, peeled and deveined

Salt and ground black pepper, as required

3 garlic cloves, minced

4 large zucchinis, spiralized with blade C

4-6 fresh basil leaves, chopped

- In a large skillet, melt the coconut oil over medium heat and sauté garlic for about 1 minute.
- Add the shrimp and cook for about 2-3 minutes.
- Add the zucchini and cook for about 2-3 minutes, tossing occasionally.
- Stir in the salt and black pepper and remove from heat.
- Serve with the garnishing of basil leaves.

Per Serving: Calories: 249; Total Fat: 9.3g; Saturated Fat: 6.6g
Protein: 29.9g; Carbs: 13.3g; Fiber: 3.6g; Sugar: 5.6g

Shrimp & Veggies Curry

Serves: 6 / Preparation time: 15 minutes / Cooking time: 15 minutes

2 teaspoons coconut oil

1½ medium white onions, sliced

2 medium green bell peppers, seeded and sliced

3 medium carrots, peeled and sliced thinly

3 garlic cloves, chopped finely

1 tablespoon fresh ginger, chopped finely

2½ teaspoons curry powder

1½ pounds shrimp, peeled and deveined

1 cup unsweetened coconut milk

2 tablespoons water

2 tablespoons fresh lime juice

Salt and ground black pepper, as required

2 tablespoons fresh cilantro, chopped

- In a large skillet, heat oil over medium-high heat and sauté the onion for about 4-5 minutes.
- Add the bell peppers and carrot and sauté for about 3-4 minutes.
- Add the garlic, ginger and curry powder and sauté for about 1 minute.
- Add the shrimp and sauté for about 1 minute.
- Stir in the coconut milk and water and cook for about 3-4 minutes, stirring occasionally.
- Stir in lime juice and remove from heat.
- Serve hot with the garnishing of cilantro.

Per Serving: Calories: 285; Total Fat: 13.3g; Saturated Fat: 10.4g
Protein: 28g; Carbs: 14.2g; Fiber: 3.2g; Sugar: 6.1g

Shrimp & Fruit Curry

Serves: 6 / Preparation time: 15 minutes / Cooking time: 12 minutes

1 tablespoon coconut oil

½ cup onion, sliced thinly

1½ pounds shrimp, peeled and deveined

½ of red bell pepper, seeded and sliced thinly

1 mango, peeled, pitted and sliced

8 ounces can of pineapple tidbits with unsweetened juice

1 cup unsweetened coconut milk

1 tablespoon red curry paste

2 tablespoons red boat fish sauce

2 tablespoons fresh cilantro, chopped

- In a skillet, melt the coconut oil over medium-high heat and sauté the onion for about 3-4 minutes.
- With a spoon, push the onion to sides of the pan.
- Add the shrimp and cook for about 2 minutes per side.
- Stir in the bell peppers and cook for about 3-4 minutes.
- Add the remaining ingredients except cilantro and simmer for about 5 minutes.
- Serve hot with the garnishing of cilantro.

Per Serving: Calories: 325; Total Fat: 14.8g; Saturated Fat: 11.3g
Protein: 28.9g; Carbs: 20.4g; Fiber: 2.4g; Sugar: 15.4g

Squid with Veggies

Serves: 4 / Preparation time: 15 minutes / Cooking time: 10 minutes

1 teaspoon olive oil

2 red bell peppers, seeded and cut into strips

¾ pound squids, cleaned

1 teaspoon fresh ginger, minced

Salt and ground black pepper, as required

2 carrots, peeled and chopped

½ of eggplant, chopped

2 tablespoons red boat fish sauce

½ teaspoon paprika

1 cup fresh spinach, chopped

- In a skillet, heat the oil over medium heat and stir fry the carrots, bell pepper and eggplant for about 3-4 minutes.
- Add the remaining ingredients except spinach and cook for about 1-2 minutes.
- Stir in the spinach and cook for about 3-4 minutes.
- Remove from the heat and serve immediately.

Per Serving: Calories: 138; Total Fat: 2.7g; Saturated Fat: 0.5g
Protein: 17g; Carbs: 14.2g; Fiber: 3.9g; Sugar: 6.3g

Lentils in Tomato Sauce

Serves: 4 / Preparation time: 10 minutes / Cooking time: 20 minutes

For Tomato Puree

1 cup tomatoes, chopped

1 garlic clove, chopped

1 (1-inch) piece fresh ginger, chopped

1 green chili, chopped

¼ cup water

For Lentils

1 cup red lentils

3 cups water

1 tablespoon olive oil

½ of medium onion, chopped finely

½ teaspoon ground cumin

½ teaspoon cayenne pepper

¼ teaspoon ground turmeric

¼ cup fresh parsley leaves, chopped

- For tomato paste: in a blender, add all ingredients and pulse until a smooth puree forms. Set aside.
- In a large pan, place 3 cups of the water and lentils over high heat and bring to a boil.
- Now, reduce the heat to medium-low and simmer, covered for about 15 minutes or until tender enough.
- Drain the lentils completely.
- Meanwhile, in a large skillet, heat the oil over medium heat and sauté the onion for about 2-3 minutes.
- Add the spices and sauté for about 1 minute.
- Add the tomato puree and cook for about 4-5 minutes, stirring continuously.
- Stir in the lentils and cook for about 4-5 minutes or until desired doneness.
- Serve hot with the garnishing of parsley.

Per Serving: Calories: 219; Total Fat: 4.3g; Saturated Fat: 0.6g
Protein: 13.2g; Carbs: 32.9g; Fiber: 15.8g; Sugar: 2.9g

Kidney Beans Chili

Serves: 3 / Preparation time: 10 minutes / Cooking time: 21 minutes

1 tablespoon olive oil

1 onion, chopped

8 ounces fresh button mushrooms, sliced

1/3 cup sun-dried tomatoes, chopped roughly

1 (15-ounce) can kidney beans

3 tablespoons homemade tomato paste

2 tablespoons red chili powder

1 tablespoon ground cumin

Salt and ground black pepper, as required

1 tablespoon fresh parsley, chopped

- In a large pan, heat the oil over medium heat and sauté the onion for about 4-5 minutes.
- Add the mushrooms and sundried tomatoes and sauté for about 5-6 minutes.
- Add the kidney beans with liquid, tomato paste, chili powder and cumin and bring to a boil.
- Reduce the heat to low and simmer for about 10 minutes.
- Stir in the salt and black pepper and remove from the heat.
- Serve hot with the garnishing of parsley.

Per Serving: Calories: 228; Total Fat: 6.4g; Saturated Fat: 0.9g
Protein: 14g; Carbs: 34.4g; Fiber: 16g; Sugar: 5.8g

Chickpeas Curry

Serves: 3 / Preparation time: 10 minutes / Cooking time: 5 minutes

2 tablespoons olive oil

2 medium onions, chopped

3 garlic cloves, chopped

1-2 teaspoons curry paste

1 (14-ounce) can unsweetened coconut milk

1 (15-ounce) can low-sodium chickpeas, rinsed and drained

1 tablespoon coconut aminos

2-3 medium tomatoes, chopped

1 cup fresh basil, chopped

1 teaspoon raw honey

1 tablespoon fresh lime juice

- In a large pan, heat the oil over medium heat and sauté the onions for about 2-3 minutes.
- Add the garlic and curry paste and sauté for about 1 minute.
- Stir in the coconut milk and cook for about 1 minute, stirring continuously.
- Stir in the chickpeas and coconut aminos and bring to a boil.
- Cook for about 1-2 minutes.
- Add the tomatoes, basil, honey and lime juice and simmer for about 2 minutes.
- Remove from the heat and serve hot.

Per Serving: Calories: 472; Total Fat: 30.5g; Saturated Fat: 18.1g
Protein: 10g; Carbs: 37.3g; Fiber: 6.7g; Sugar: 11.1g

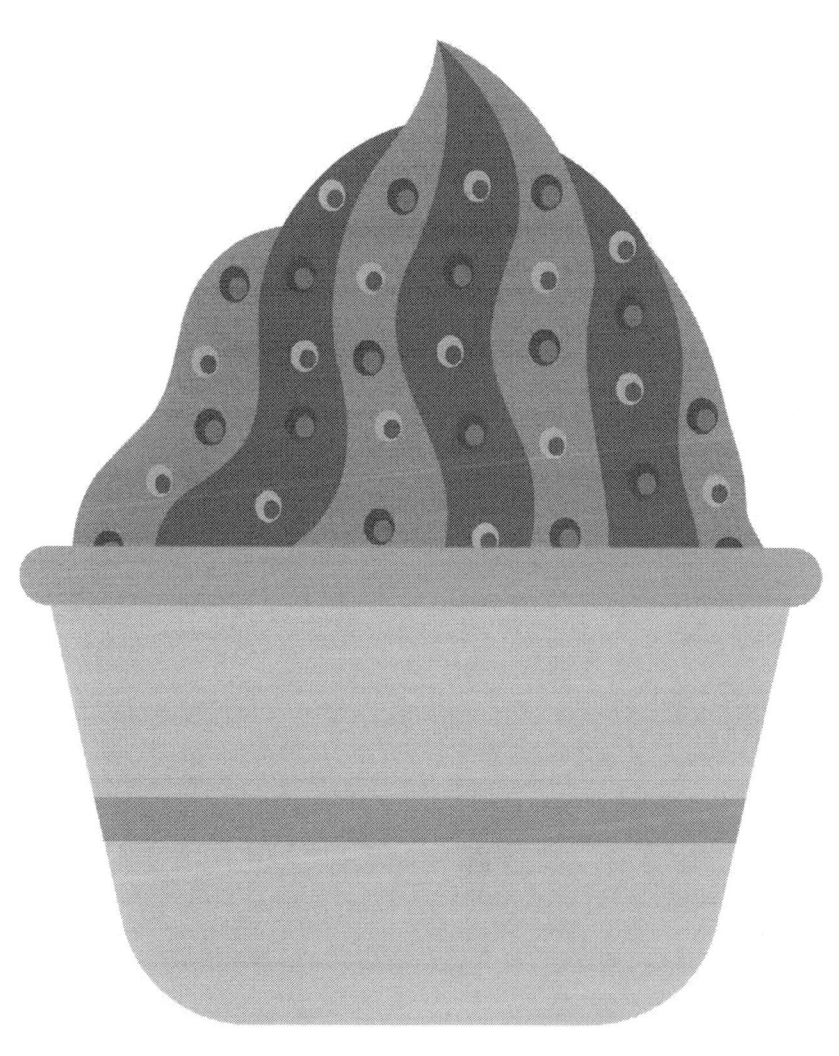

DESSERT RECIPES

Contents

Strawberry Ice Cream

Serves: 4 / Preparation time: 15 minutes

1 cup fresh strawberries, hulled and sliced   ½ small banana, peeled and sliced

2 tablespoon unsweetened coconut, shredded   ½ cup coconut cream

- In a powerful blender, add all ingredients and pulse until smooth.
- Transfer into an ice cream maker and process according to manufacturer's directions.
- Now, transfer into an airtight container and freeze for at least 3 to 4 hours, stirring after every 30 minutes.

Per Serving: Calories: 101; Total Fat: 8.1g; Saturated Fat: 7.1g
Protein: 1.2g; Carbs: 7.7g; Fiber: 1.9g; Sugar: 4.5g

Mango Sorbet

Serves: 8 / Preparation time: 10 minutes

3 cups frozen mango, peeled, pitted and chopped

10 fresh mint leaves

2 tablespoons fresh lime juice

½ cup chilled water

- In a powerful blender, add all ingredients and pulse until smooth.
- Transfer into serving bowls and serve immediately.

Per Serving: Calories: 38; Total Fat: 0.3g; Saturated Fat: 0.1g
Protein: 0.6g; Carbs: 9.4g; Fiber: 1.1g; Sugar: 8.5g

Chocolate Mousse

Serves: 4 / Preparation time: 10 minutes

½ cup unsweetened almond milk

4 Medjool dates, pitted and chopped

2 tablespoons cacao powder

2 tablespoons fresh raspberries

1 cup cooked black beans

½ cup walnuts, chopped

1 teaspoon organic vanilla extract

4 fresh mint leaves

- In a food processor, add all ingredients and pulse until smooth and creamy.
- Transfer into serving bowls and refrigerate to chill before serving.
- Garnish with raspberries and mint leaves and serve.

Per Serving: Calories: 342; Total Fat: 11g; Saturated Fat: 1.1g
Protein: 15.5g; Carbs: 50.8g; Fiber: 11.4g; Sugar: 15.8g

Berries Pudding

Serves: 3 / Preparation time: 10 minutes

2 tablespoons raw hemp seeds, shelled

2 ripe bananas, peeled

1-3 tablespoons maple syrup

1/8 teaspoon ground cinnamon

2 cups fresh mixed berries

2 tablespoons unsweetened coconut milk

2 tablespoons chia seeds

- In a food processor, add the berries, bananas and coconut milk and pulse until well combined.
- Add the maple syrup and pulse until well combined.
- Add the hemp seeds, chia seeds and cinnamon and pulse until well combined.
- Transfer the pudding into a serving bowl.
- Cover the bowl and refrigerate to chill for at least 2 hours before serving.

Per Serving: Calories: 223; Total Fat: 7.8g; Saturated Fat: 2.7g
Protein: 5g; Carbs: 36.8g; Fiber: 7.8g; Sugar: 20.6g

Chocolaty Beans Brownies

Serves: 12 / Preparation time: 15 minutes / Cooking time: 30 minutes

2 cups cooked black beans

2 tablespoon organic vanilla extract

1 tablespoon ground cinnamon

12 Medjool dates, pitted and chopped

¼ cup cacao powder

- Preheat the oven to 350 degrees F. Line a large baking dish with parchment paper.
- In a food processor, add all ingredients except cacao powder and cinnamon and pulse till well combined and smooth.
- Transfer the mixture into a large bowl.
- Add the cacao powder and cinnamon and stir to combine.
- Now, transfer the mixture into prepared baking dish and with the back of a spatula, smooth the top surface.
- Bake for about 30 minutes.
- Remove from oven and let it cool.
- With a sharp knife cut into 12 equal-sized brownies and serve.

Per Serving: Calories: 178; Total Fat: 0.9g; Saturated Fat: 0.3g
Protein: 7.8g; Carbs: 36.7g; Fiber: 7.3g; Sugar: 13.6g

Chocolate Mug Cake

Serves: 1 / Preparation time: 5 minutes / Cooking time: 2 minutes

¼ cup almond flour

Salt, as required

½ teaspoon organic vanilla extract

¼ teaspoon ground cinnamon

1 large organic egg

¼ cup banana, peeled and mashed

1-2 tablespoons 70% unsweetened mini chocolate chips

- Grease a microwave-safe mug.
- In a bowl, mix together flour, cinnamon and salt.
- In another small bowl, add the egg and vanilla and beat well.
- Add the banana and beat well.
- Add the egg mixture into flour mixture and mix until just combined.
- Gently, fold in the chocolate chips.
- Transfer the mixture into prepared mug and microwave on High for about 2 minutes.
- Remove from microwave and set aside to cool for about 5 minutes before serving.

Per Serving: Calories: 392; Total Fat: 28.1g; Saturated Fat: 7.6g
Protein: 8.7g; Carbs: 18.7g; Fiber: 6.3g; Sugar: 6.3g

Strawberry Cake

Serves: 10 / Preparation time: 20 minutes / Cooking time: 35 minutes

For Cake
2 cups almond flour
½ cup arrowroot powder
Pinch of salt
½ cup raw honey
1 tablespoon organic vanilla extract
For Frosting
¾ cup freeze-dried strawberries
1/3 cup raw honey
2 tablespoons coconut flour
Fresh strawberries, hulled and sliced (as required)

½ cup coconut flour
2 teaspoons baking soda
1 cup unsweetened applesauce
9 organic eggs
2 teaspoons apple cider vinegar

1½ cups coconut oil, softened
¼ cup arrowroot powder

- Preheat the oven to 325 degrees F. Grease 2 (9-inch) round cake pans.
- For cake: in a large bowl, mix together flours, arrowroot, baking soda and salt.
- In another bowl, add applesauce, honey, eggs, vanilla extract and vinegar and beat until well combined.
- Add the egg mixture into flour mixture and mix until well combined.
- Divide the mixture into prepared cake pans evenly.
- Bake for about 25-35 minutes or until a toothpick inserted in the center comes out clean.
- Remove from oven and place the pans onto wire rack to cool for about 10 minutes.
- Carefully invert the cakes onto the wire rack to cool completely.
- Meanwhile, for frosting: in a coffee grinder, add dried strawberries and pulse until powdered.
- Through a fine strainer, strain the strawberry powder.
- In a bowl, add remaining ingredients except fresh strawberries and beat until smooth.
- Slowly, add strawberry powder, beating continuously until well combined.
- Arrange one cake onto a platter and spread the strawberry mixture on top.
- Place the second cake on top.
- Now, spread the frosting over the cake.
- Cut into desired sized slices and serve.

Per Serving: Calories: 638; Total Fat: 48.8g; Saturated Fat: 30.4g
Protein: 5.4g; Carbs: 43.1g; Fiber: 3.4g; Sugar: 29g

Apple Crisp

Serves: 4 / Preparation time: 15 minutes / Cooking time: 20 minutes

For Filling

2 large apples, peeled, cored and chopped

2 tablespoons water

2 tablespoons fresh apple juice

¼ teaspoon ground cinnamon

For Topping

½ cup quick rolled oats

2 tablespoons walnuts, chopped

¼ cup water

¼ cup unsweetened coconut flakes

½ teaspoon ground cinnamon

- Preheat the oven to 300 degrees F.
- For filling: in a baking dish, place all the ingredients and gently mix.
- For topping in a bowl, add all the ingredients and mix well.
- Spread the topping over filling mixture evenly.
- Bake for about 20 minutes or until top becomes golden brown.
- Serve warm.

Per Serving: Calories: 201; Total Fat: 4.9g; Saturated Fat: 1.6g
Protein: 3.4g; Carbs: 38.2g; Fiber: 5g; Sugar: 23.9g

Banana Crumb

Serves: 2 / Preparation time: 10 minutes / Cooking time: 25 minutes

¼ cup coconut, shredded

1 tablespoon fresh lemon juice

Pinch of ground cinnamon

3 tablespoons coconut oil, melted

¼ teaspoon organic vanilla extract

2 medium bananas, peeled and sliced

- Preheat the oven to 350 degrees F. Lightly, grease 2 ramekins.
- In a bowl, add all ingredients except bananas and mix well.
- In the bottom of the prepared ramekins, place the banana slices in and top with coconut mixture evenly.
- Bake for about 25 minutes or until top becomes golden brown.
- Serve warm.

Per Serving: Calories: 320; Total Fat: 24.2g; Saturated Fat: 20.8g
Protein: 1.7g; Carbs: 28.8g; Fiber: 4.1g; Sugar: 15.3g

Blueberry Crumble

Serves: 4 / Preparation time: 15 minutes / Cooking time: 40 minutes

¼ cup coconut flour

¼ cup arrowroot flour

¾ teaspoon baking soda

¼ cup banana, peeled and mashed

2 tablespoons coconut oil, melted

3 tablespoons filtered water

½ tablespoon fresh lemon juice

1½ cups fresh blueberries

- Preheat the oven to 300 degrees F. Lightly, grease an 8x8-inch baking dish.
- In a large bowl, add all the ingredients except blueberries and mix well.
- In the bottom of prepared baking dish, place blueberries evenly and top with flour mixture.
- Bake for about 35-40 minutes or until top becomes golden brown.

Per Serving: Calories: 107; Total Fat: 7.2g; Saturated Fat: 6g
Protein: 1g; Carbs: 11.6g; Fiber: 2g; Sugar: 6.7g

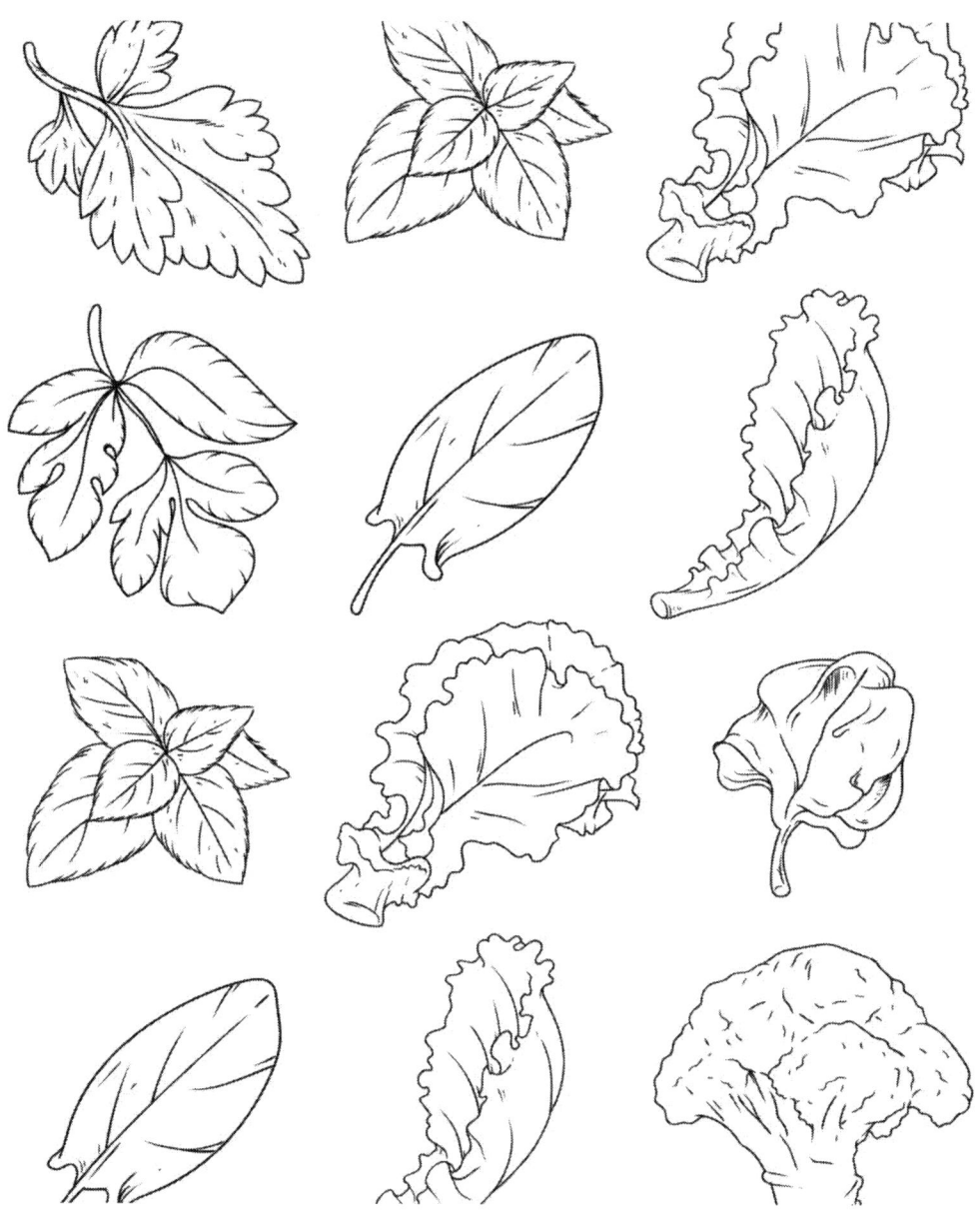

THE "DIRTY DOZEN" AND "CLEAN 15"

Every year, the Environmental Working Group releases a list of the produce with the most pesticide residue (Dirty Dozen) and a list of the ones with the least **chance of having residue (Clean 15). It's based on analysis from the U.S.** Department of Agriculture Pesticide Data Program report.

The Environmental Working Group found that 70% of the 48 types of produce tested had residues of at least one type of pesticide. In total there were 178 different pesticides and pesticide breakdown products. This residue can stay on veggies and fruit even after they are washed and peeled. All pesticides are toxic to humans and consuming them can cause damage to the nervous system, reproductive system, cancer, a weakened immune system, and more. Women who are pregnant can expose their unborn children to toxins through their diet, and continued exposure to pesticides can affect their development.

This info can help you choose the best fruits and veggies, as well as which ones you should always try to buy organic.

The Dirty Dozen

- Strawberries
- Spinach
- Nectarines
- Apples
- Peaches
- Celery
- Grapes
- Pears
- Cherries
- Tomatoes
- Sweet bell peppers
- Potatoes

The Clean 15

- Sweet corn
- Avocados
- Pineapples
- Cabbage
- Onions
- Frozen sweet peas
- Papayas
- Asparagus
- Mangoes
- Eggplant
- Honeydew
- Kiwi
- Cantaloupe
- Cauliflower
- Grapefruit

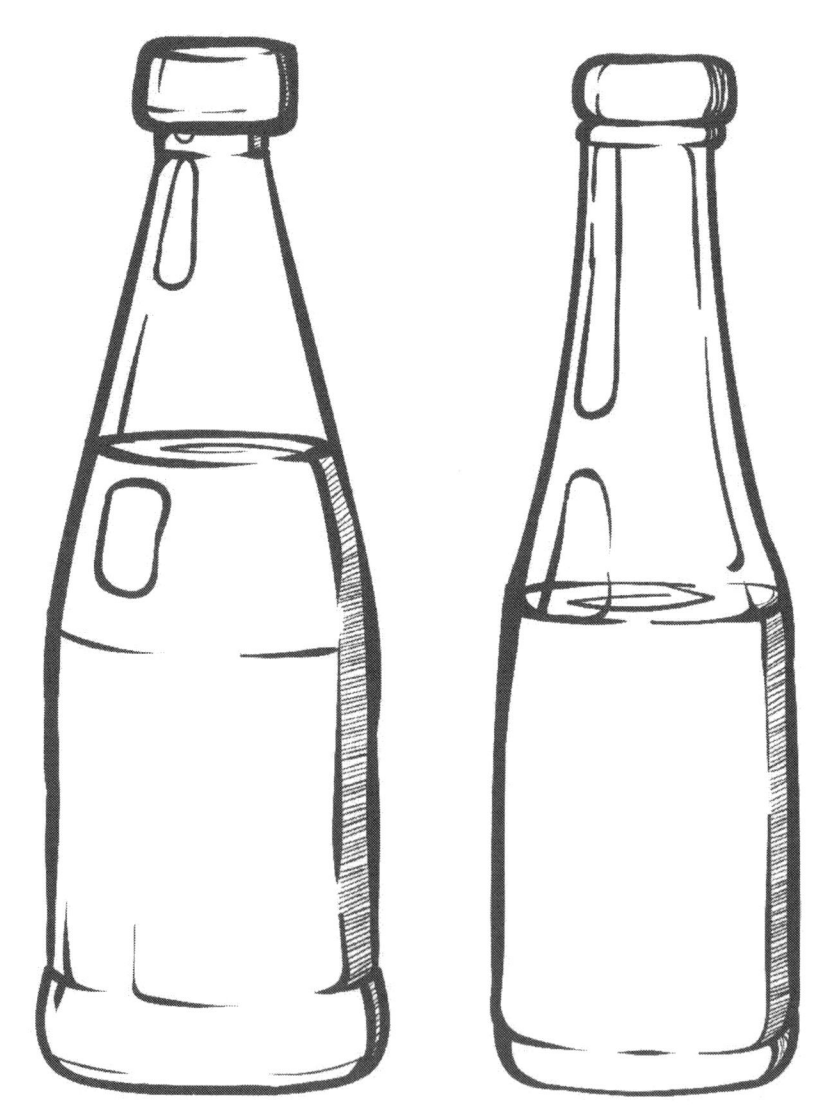

MEASUREMENT CONVERSION TABLES

Volume Equivalents (Dry)

US Standard	Metric (Approx.)
¼ teaspoon	1 ml
½ teaspoon	2 ml
1 teaspoon	5 ml
1 tablespoon	15 ml
¼ cup	59 ml
½ cup	118 ml
1 cup	235 ml

Weight Equivalents

US Standard	Metric (Approx.)
½ ounce	15 g
1 ounce	30 g
2 ounces	60 g
4 ounces	115 g
8 ounces	225 g
12 ounces	340 g
16 oz or 1 lb	455 g

Volume Equivalents (Liquid)

US Standard	US Standard (ounces)	Metric (Approx.)
2 tablespoons	1 fl oz	30 ml
¼ cup	2 fl oz	60 ml
½ cup	4 fl oz	120 ml
1 cup	8 fl oz	240 ml
1 ½ cups	12 fl oz	355 ml
2 cups or 1 pint	16 fl oz	475 ml
4 cups or 1 quart	32 fl oz	1 L
1 gallon	128 fl oz	4 L

Oven Temperatures

Fahrenheit (F)	Celsius (C) (Approx)
250°F	120°C
300°F	150°C
325°F	165°C
350°F	180°C
375°F	190°C
400°F	200°C
425°F	220°C
450°F	230°C

INDEX

30 DAY MEAL PLAN

DAY	BREAKFAST	LUNCH	DINNER
1	Zucchini with Eggs 47	Shrimp Kabobs 74	Pan Seared Lamb Chops 105
2	Blueberry Pancakes 35	Turkey & Apple Burgers 67	Glazed Chicken Thighs 93
3	Oats & Fruit Smoothie Bowl 26	Broccoli Soup 59	Beef & Plum Salad 85
4	Banana Bread 40	Oats & Black Beans Burgers 64	Stuffed Turkey Breast 98
5	Quinoa & Orange Porridge 32	Cabbage with Apple 78	Shrimp & Veggies Curry 108
6	Apple Smoothie 22	Zoodles & Radish Salad 54	Beef & Veggie Stew 89
7	Herbed Tomato Frittata 44	Veggie Kabobs 73	Beef with Lentils 101
8	Egg White Waffles 34	Sweet & Sour Shrimp 80	Glazed Flank Steak 99
9	Overnight Oatmeal 31	Meatballs with Apple Chutney 61	Squid with Veggies 110
10	Fruity Chia Seed Pudding 28	Kale with Cranberries 79	Grilled Chicken Breast 94
11	Chicken & Veggie Casserole 45	Chicken & Veggie Kabobs 72	Shrimp & Fruit Curry 109
12	Zucchini Bread 39	Quinoa & Mango Salad 56	Quinoa Soup 88
13	Chia Seed Pudding 27	Quinoa with Green Peas 81	Chicken with Fruit & Veggies 96
14	Orange & Carrot Juice 20	Veggie Meatballs 63	Broiled Lamb Shoulder 104
15	Veggies Quiche 46	Broccoli & Carrot Salad 53	Lamb Chili 92
16	Caraway Seed Bread 41	Spinach in Creamy Sauce 76	Lentils in Tomato Sauce 111
17	Pumpkin Muffins 37	Egg Drop Soup 58	Chicken & Broccoli Casserole 97

18	Fruit & Greens Smoothie 24	Veggies Burgers 68	Poached Salmon 106
19	Quinoa & Coconut Granola 49	Broccoli with Kale 77	Chicken Salad 84
20	Green Fruit Juice 21	Black Beans Meatballs 62	Ground Beef with Peas 102
21	Apple Omelet 43	Chilled Zucchini Soup 57	Beef Chili 91
22	Vanilla Crepes 33	Turkey & Beans Lettuce Wraps 69	Kidney Beans Chili 112
23	Eggs in Avocado Cups 42	Shrimp & Watermelon Kabobs 75	Shrimp with Zoodles 107
24	Fruit Cocktail 25	Shrimp Lettuce Wraps 70	Chicken & Zucchini Soup 87
25	Apple Porridge 29	Pumpkin Soup 60	Chicken Chili 90
26	Chicken & Zucchini Pancakes 36	Greens Salad 55	Stuffed Bell Peppers 103
27	Sweet Potato & Bell Pepper Hash 48	Beef & Veggie Burgers 66	Chicken with Pineapple & Bell Peppers 95
28	Banana & Date Smoothie 23	Chicken & Pineapple Kabobs 71	Chickpeas Curry 113
29	Banana Porridge 30	Beet & Orange Salad 52	Beef with Cauliflower 100
30	Chicken & Veggie Muffins 38	Salmon & Quinoa Burgers 65	Salmon & Veggie Salad 86

Manufactured by Amazon.ca
Bolton, ON

21749278R00074